What a Pain

A Doctor's Guide to Understanding and Treating Pain

by Gary Saff MD

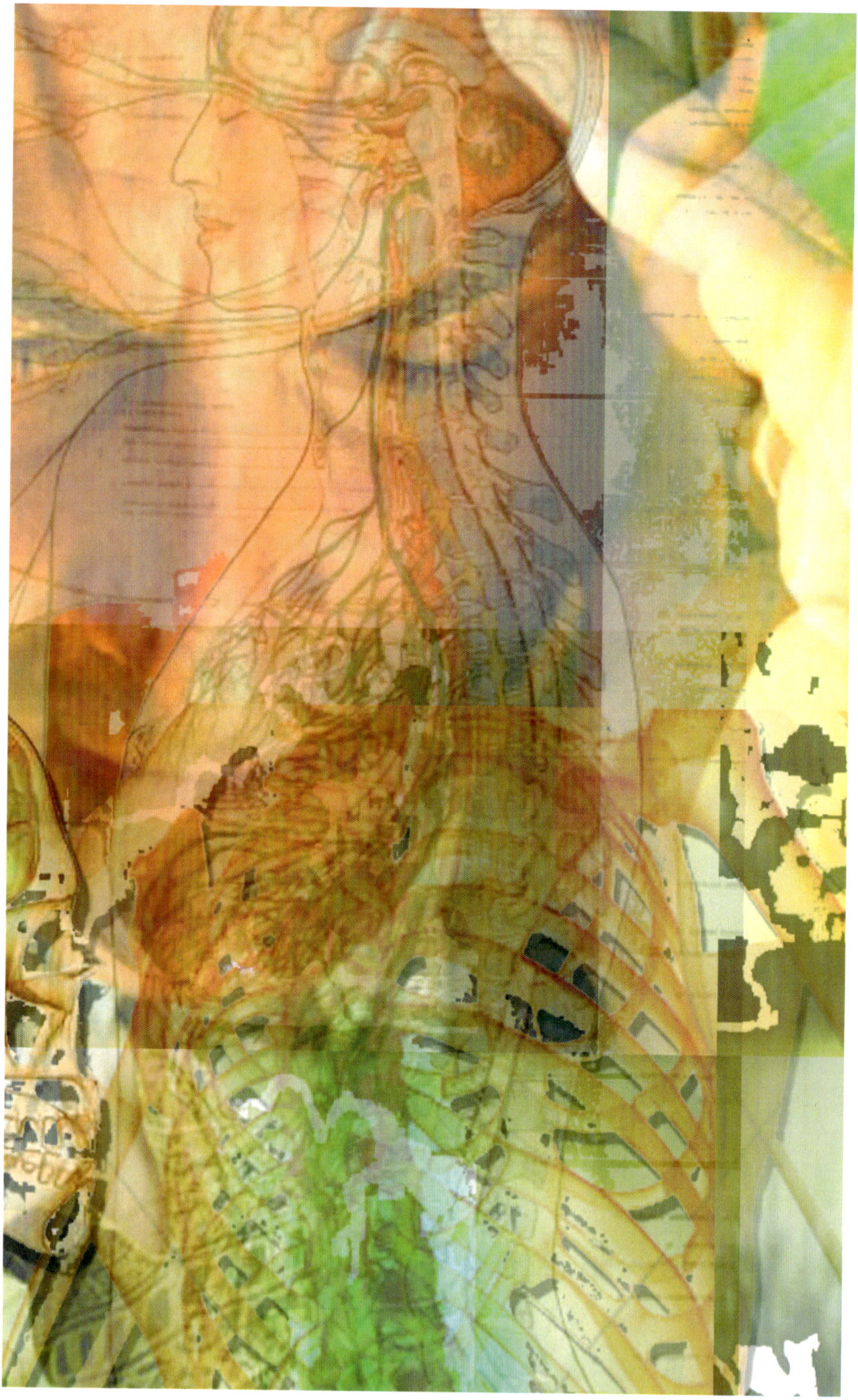

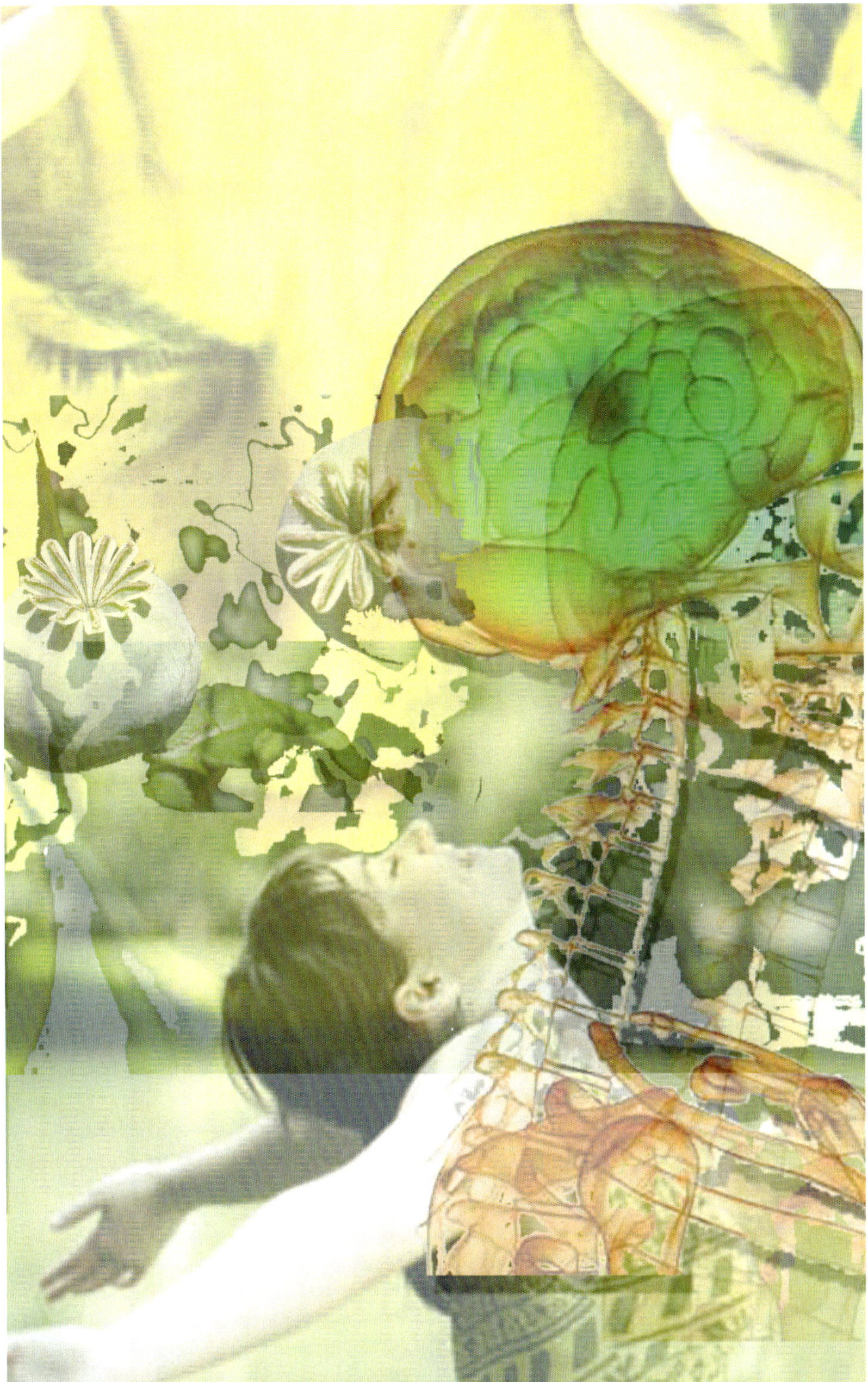

ISBN #: 978-0-9624333-7-5

BG Publishing International Ft. Lauderdale

Acknowledgements

I'd like to acknowledge colleagues for their assistance: Lisa Saff Koche, M.D., alternative medicine specialist at Spectra Complete, Tampa, Florida; Luis Mejia, MA, PT, of Mejia Physical Therapy and Wellness in Weston, Florida; Noel Wallis, insurance advisor for Wallis Financial Group in Lake Worth, Florida; Sheila Danzig for her brilliant ideas, emails, and encouragement; Ruth Saff for her editing skills.

I also want to acknowledge my patients, both past, present, and future, who continue to be my greatest teachers in understanding the specialty of pain management.

Dedication

This book is dedicated to Tamara, my cherished wife, along with our 3 beloved children, Julia, Jenna and Evan. Their love and support make my life complete. Dedication also goes to my parents, Harvey and Myra Saff, and to the memory of my grandparents being my first patients, Rose and Irving Saff, Nettie and Milton Rosen. Collectively they have instilled in me the desire for knowledge and education along with the confidence to follow my dreams and help others in my medical career.

About the Author

Dr. Gary Saff of Integrated Pain Solutions of South Florida is an M.D. trained native of South Florida where he currently practices as an interventional pain management specialist. Ivy League trained, he did his pain management fellowship at Memorial Sloan-Kettering Cancer Center. More recently, he was the director of pain management services at Cleveland Clinic and formerly a director at Columbia University's St. Lukes-Roosevelt Hospital. He is licensed with the American Board of Anesthesiology, the American Society of Pain Management and is also licensed in acupuncture. He has spent time in the Amazon jungle learning medicine from shamans as well as spending time learning Eastern medicine and acupuncture techniques. He has published many articles and has given lectures both nationally and internationally. He can be contacted through his practice, Integrated Pain Solutions of South Florida at 954-772-7552 or via the web at http://www.ipssf.com.

Table of Contents

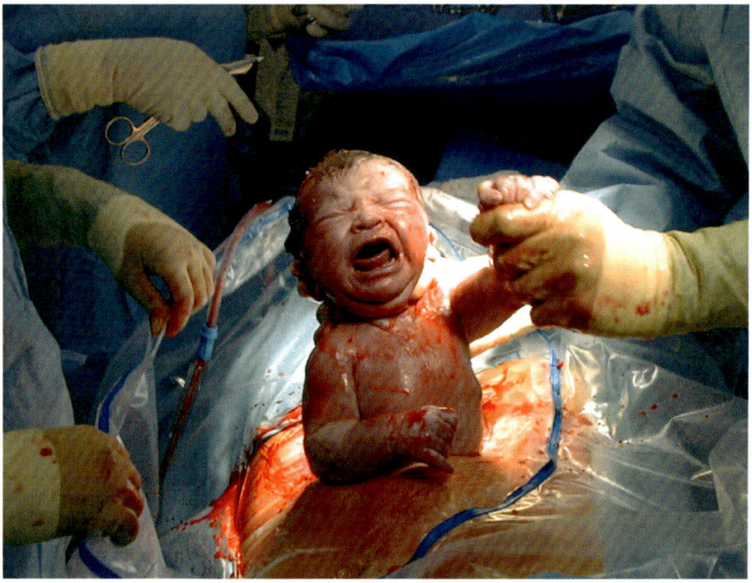

CHAPTER 1
In the Beginning

The tiny creation began to tremble, as the sharp blast of cold air penetrated the tender, moist warmth surrounding him. A piercing, primal scream filled the air and the infant's face twisted into a grimace. This very first physical sensation for this new human being permeated all his senses as his new life began. The first sensation for all of us, the exact moment we're born, is that of PAIN.

Life in the womb is sheltered and we are nurtured in a lovely, quiet place, lulled by endless comforting rhythms and undulations. The sight of tremulous sunset colors is resplendent in our mother's womb, our safe home for many months. Occasionally we are conscious of pleasant sounds, and we turn our tiny heads toward the music or the calming voices and then we return to sleep – and grow stronger.

Birth is not a pleasant feeling for the baby entering this world. When the time comes for our entrance, we are submitted to a terrifying sequence of events. Our entire body is compressed to the point of near suffocation. Forces of creation push us downward and outward into a glaring environment. We burst into a fiercely dry environment in which our lungs strain to function. Our first human contact is by a strong arm in a sterile surgical gown, tightly wrapping us in coarse cloth, before being handed off for measurements and tests that make us scream even louder. The undulations become staccato and cacophonous. We are furious, and we scream in horrible fear and pain. This is the pain that many of us remember, at a subliminal level for the remainder of our lives. It can create a behavior that drives us to always seek to regain the nurturing comfort of the womb. No wonder we are by nature, very afraid of pain.

Pain is the first alarm warning us of danger. People who are born without the blessing of feeling pain are always in serious trouble; they can't avoid what they can't intuit through one of their senses. We get too close to a flame and the heat causes us to flinch and pull back, saving us from serious burns. A child cuts his finger on a sharp object and pulls away, avoiding a deeper cut. A skinned knee helps a child learn how to balance more carefully on a skateboard, or ride his or her first bike. This kind of pain - the acute kind - is present for a reason: to warn us of danger. Or perhaps, acute pain will draw our attention to a condition needing our attention, such as infection from an appendix about to rupture! PAIN is invaluable, and we should be humbly grateful every single time we experience the sensation of pain.

Chronic pain, however, is a different story. Of what human value is chronic pain? Some might consider chronic pain as a tedious, drawn-out warning of mild to severe danger. Chronic pain is ongoing discomfort of varying degrees - from the kind of pain that can almost be ignored to the biting, encompassing pain that simply dominates the conscious mind. The development of chronic pain should never be ignored. Usually, if not always, pain needs the careful consideration of a qualified physician in order to remedy the situation before it controls the patient's life.

Nothing is as discouraging or as depressing as the feeling of uselessness, helplessness and depression from unrelieved pain. The victim is left lonely and afraid. We are basically social beings, and as long as we can relate to each other and help someone else occasionally (even if it's just with a smile of encouragement), we feel better physically and mentally. However, when chronic pain dominates our lives, all the small interactions that make us smile and laugh as humans is washed away.

Our brief time in *utero* is a miniature mirror image of the stages of human development, an indisputable fact many feel is another testimony to the evidence of either a phenomenal coincidence or power to control our destinies. First year medical students are mostly uninspired and prefer to focus on "just the facts" when it comes to skeletal structure and the organs protected in the intricate cage of our ribs that are supported by other bones connected to each other by the magic of creation and evolution. However, by the time these students reach their final year, they have attained a level of humility in the face of the level of creation about which they are learning. They have become privy to the wonders of the human skeleton and to the secret of life itself.

Most of us take our anatomy – including our skeletons – for granted, which is a very big mistake. However, this is part of our human nature and we can easily forgive ourselves as long as, at one time or another, we show our deep appreciation for the amazing attention paid to the smallest details of our physical make-up. Our minute network of nerves is the prime example of exacting details with nothing left to chance. The peripheral nervous system is exactly what its name implies: it is the system of nerves located outside the brain and spinal cord, in the peripherals of the body. The peripheral nervous system, unlike the highly condensed central nervous system, is not protected at all by the blood-brain barrier or by bones. It is constantly feeding information to the central nervous system. The "autonomic nervous system" functions to maintain bodily homeostasis and only triggers our conscious minds when something is seriously going wrong. It is a sensitive nerve interplay that conducts the first alarm of pain to the brain, experienced when we incur a wound, a symptom of disease, or an internal injury that needs attention. The reactions of the nerves are literally instantaneous. However, often in severe injuries, no pain is felt at first. This could be nature's way of letting the human mind prepare itself for the onslaught of agony to come.

For our purpose in discussing pain, think of the brain as the clearing-house in a gigantic import-export company.

Our brains have the uncanny ability to categorize the nerve impulses pulsing through our systems faster than we can have the words to describe what part of our body is injured. The brain is the epicenter where emergency procedures are assigned, administered and monitored. The brain analyzes the pain and signals us to faint, scream, or grit our teeth and wait. And, when possible, to try and stem the flow of blood, or get into a more comfortable position, or tear a shirt with our good hand and our teeth, or signal for help from a passer-by – or, in other words, to fight. Our natural instincts move into action when we are injured and we fight hard to survive. Without this survival instinct, we wouldn't make it. It is this mysterious power that makes the maimed and crippled soldiers determined to walk again, even when they have lost one or both legs and even one or both arms as well, or the young man blinded by shrapnel determined to learn Braille. The human body, under the direction of the human brain, is a tough customer. By optimizing pain management through the considerate and compassionate care of a medical professional, the patient can attain as productive a life as possible, thereby allowing for a greater quality of life and goal attainment.

Nervous System

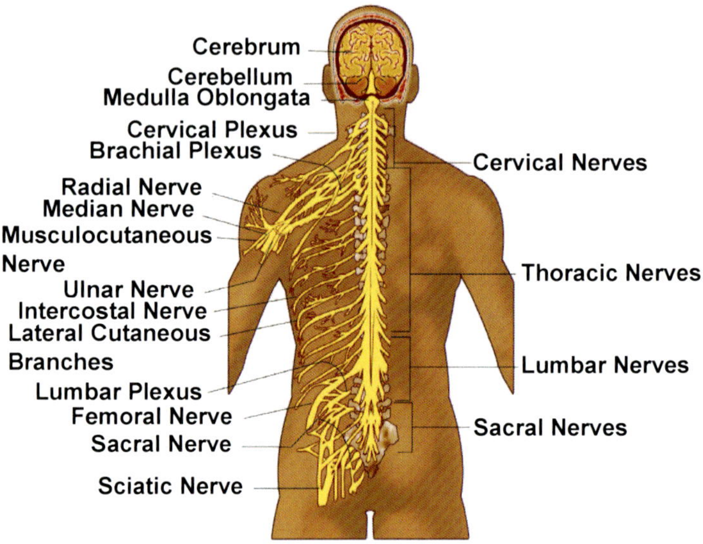

CHAPTER 2

The Nervous System and Spine

To start talking about pain, and to understand it, we must start at a focal beginning. A discussion of the nervous system and spine is a reasonable first step. If pain is present, it had to start somewhere. There had to have been an origin and a cause: a broken bone, a deep cut, a virulent infection – something gone amiss in the system. The network of nerves picks up on the lightning flashes of pain signals and alerts the brain to get ready to fight. A distinctive set of clinical symptoms are presented by different clinical conditions depending upon the location and the area in which the pain is centered. The purpose of this book is to help the patient suffering from pain to learn why pain may exist, and how to manage and deal with it on an everyday basis.

Anatomy of Nervous System

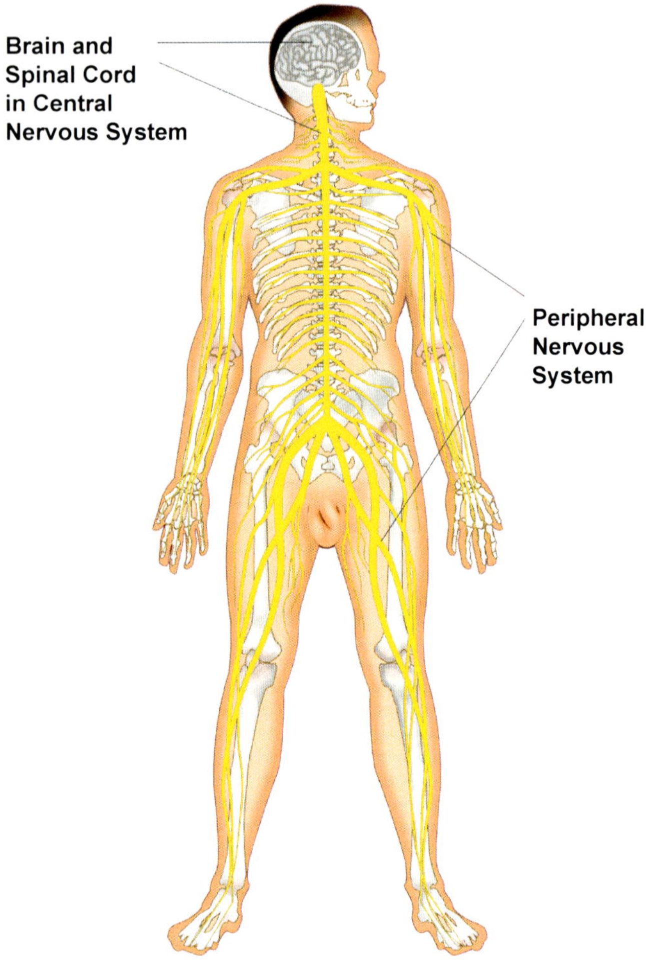

All the body's communications occur through the nervous system. The nervous system is essentially the body's electrical system which uses electrolytes, mostly sodium and potassium, to send electrical currents throughout your body. The nervous system can be easily viewed as three separate components, all of which cohesively interact together. The central nervous system (CNS) contains the brain and spinal cord. The peripheral nervous system (PNS) contains all the spinal nerves exiting from the spinal cord. Finally, the third part of the nervous system is the autonomic nervous system (ANS) which controls, unconsciously, all the vital organs. The ANS controls blood pressure, heart rate, bowel and bladder function, thermoregulation and digestion.

The brain is the "master computer processor" of all nervous system inputs, and therefore - due to its critical role - is well protected by the bony skull. It controls the ability to independently think, move, display emotion, and have volition of action. The spinal cord can be viewed as a large, ropey telephone cable, descending from the base of the brain, consisting of a myriad of smaller fibers, each fiber carrying unique information from the brain to the periphery, or sending signals to the brain from the periphery. The spinal cord extends to as low as the second lumbar vertebral level, commonly called "L2", at which point it stops and individual nerve roots filter down lower and exit out of the spinal column to the legs and sacral structures.

To an extent, the brain has the ability to autoregulate inputs. For example, the intensity of a bad smell when you step into a room may quickly fade and no longer be annoying after several minutes due to brain regulatory factors. Likewise, the spinal cord can function independently of the brain. The best example of this is the reflexes. When you step on a sharp object, the intense pain signal travels up to the spinal cord, which, in turn, automatically sends a "motor" signal to that leg to withdraw, and another to the opposite leg to give support. This happens in a split second, and the brain is notified of the event often after the action has been completed.

Spinal Cord and Nerve Roots

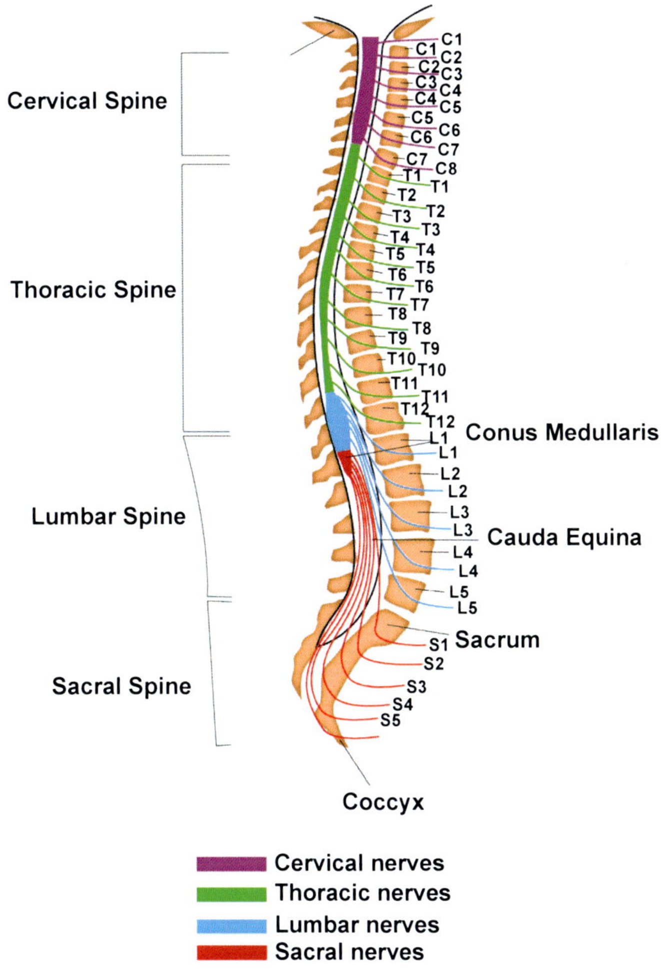

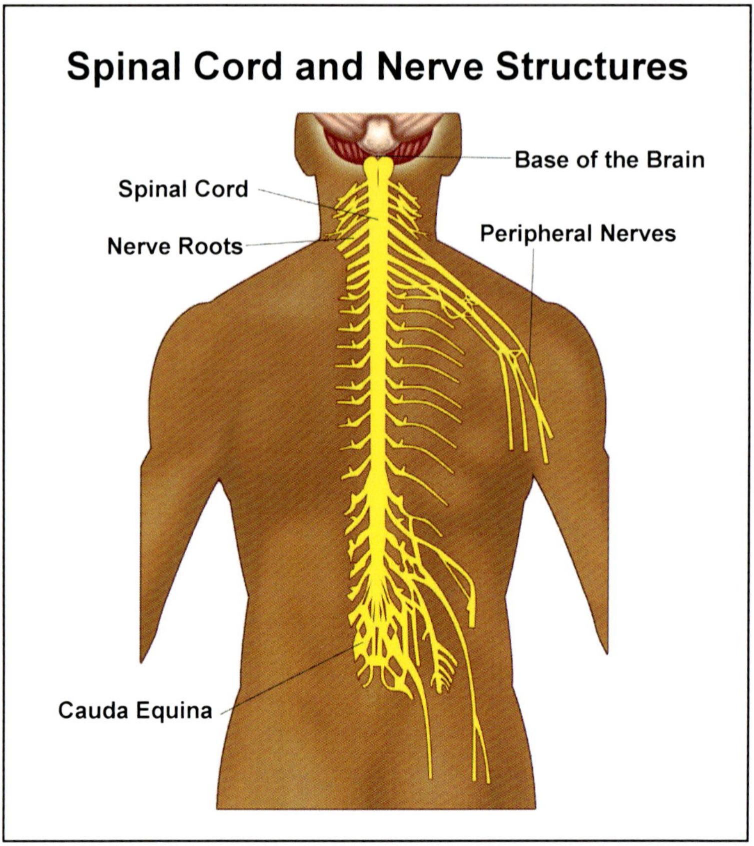

The peripheral nerves exit from the spinal cord then peel out of the vertebral column at each level, before coursing out to the periphery. Peripheral nerves have sensory functions, motor functions, or a combination of both. They may interconnect to each other very much like electrical extension cords interconnect. These connections are called "synapses" and can be the target of disease processes, causing neurological deterioration such as myasthenia gravis. The sensory nerves have receptors on the very tips which serve to collect information to send up to the central nervous system. These receptors may register various things such as temperature changes, pain, movement and stretch. The stretch receptors are triggered when, for example, a reflex hammer hits your knee (patella) tendon. The spinal cord reaction is to send a motor response to raise the leg, hence minimizing this sudden stretch to the tendon. Pain from activation of these peripheral nervous system receptors is not vague, but very well localized, much like the sensation of a knife cutting your skin. The motor nerves only target various select muscles. Therefore, when they are transected, permanent weakness can occur. The cranial nerves act similarly to the nerves coming off the spinal cord. The difference is that they join the central nervous system higher up in the brainstem.

The autonomic nervous system is comprised of a large network of small fibers that exit the CNS and diffusely spread throughout the body, and involves the internal organs as well as blood vessels and the skin. This is the "autopilot" which keeps everything regulated and on course, without you being consciously aware of it, unless things get significantly out of kilter. An example of the latter would be your awareness of labored breathing with excessive exercise, making you conscious of the fact that you need to slow down.

Autonomic Nervous System - Innervation Throughout Body

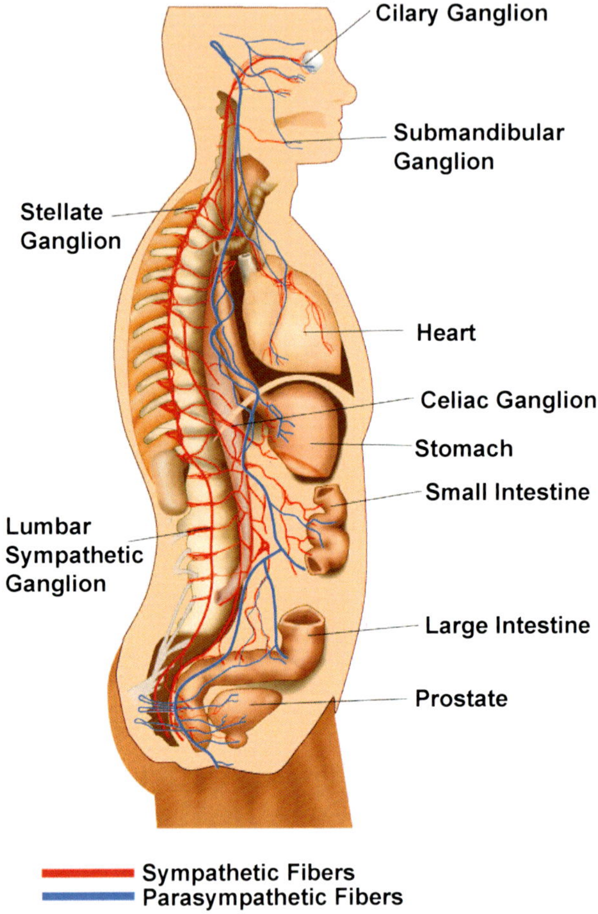

The autonomic fibers clump together in nerve bundles, called "ganglion" located in various parts of the body. An autonomic sympathetic block targets these ganglia. As the autonomic fibers exit the ganglion to the periphery, they become very "lazy" in the sense that they do not make their own neurological pathways. Instead, they ride "piggy-back" along the blood vessels or along the PNS before jumping off at their destination. Pain or irritation from the internal organs travels along the autonomic nervous system, and is brought to consciousness as a very vague, nonspecific "dis-ease," more so than true pain. Examples would be feelings of constipation or bloating. This stands in direct contrast to the well-localizing pain of the peripheral nervous system, such as being cut by a knife.

There are two main divisions in the ANS: the sympathetic and parasympathetic. The sympathetic fibers are typically known as the "fight or flight" fibers that are responsible for your body's reaction when scared or threatened. They increase your heart rate, sharpen your vision, and shunt blood to muscles in readiness for action. On the contrary, the parasympathetic nervous system is known for "rest and digest". These fibers slow down your heart rate, shunt blood to the digestive system and away from muscles, and are in full gear when you are relaxing.

Cross-section of Spine

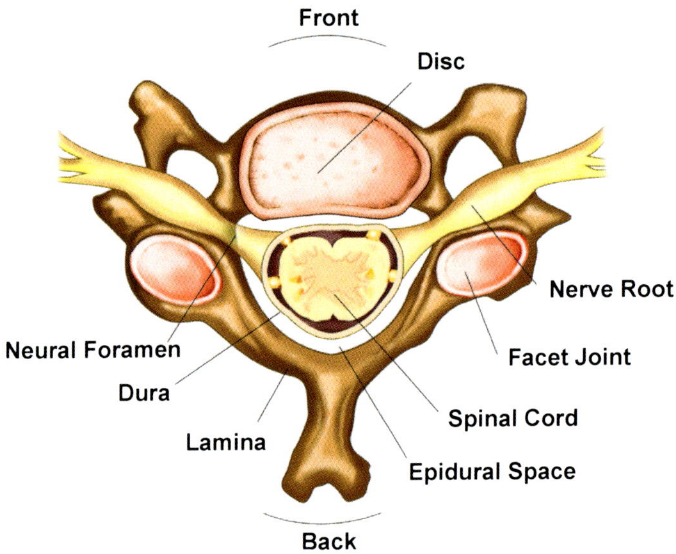

The Spine

The spine is a design of engineering genius. It functions as the bony system, which serves to support and protect the fragile nerves, much as the struts in a building serve to support and attach the electrical wiring as they pass along their way. The spine provides a safe passageway for nerves leading from every muscle, tendon, organ, and blood vessel to the brain itself. The spine is a column of interconnected bones, each separated by a disc, which starts at the base of the skull and terminates lower down in the sacral area. Starting at the top, there are seven cervical vertebrae, followed by twelve thoracic, and then five lumbar vertebrae. This is true with mammals; even a giraffe has only seven cervical vertebrae in its long neck.

Lumbar Spine - Side View

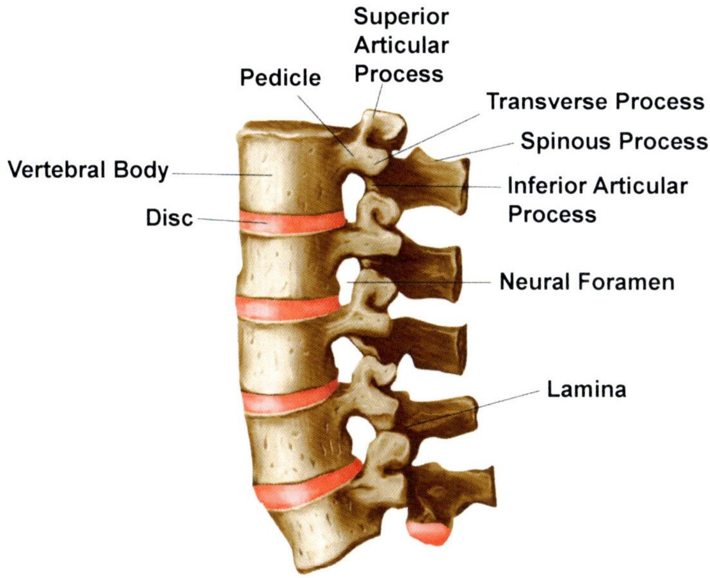

The majority of motion in the spine comes from movement in the disc spaces between the vertebral bodies of the lower part of the cervical and lower part of the lumbar vertebrae. By design, there is little motion of the thoracic vertebrae which connect in the front to the rib cage, hence protecting vital internal organs from torsion. Where one has motion in these lower cervical and lumbar segments, there also will be more advanced degeneration, both of the discs, as well as of the vertebral bodies.

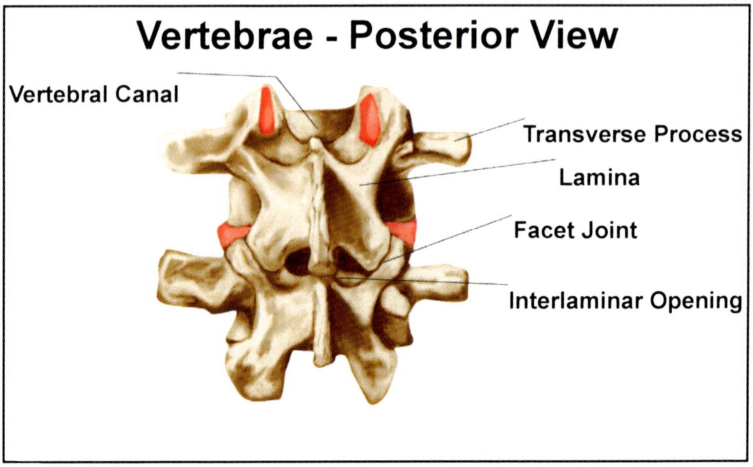

Within the bony vertebral body, and protected by it, is the spinal canal. Housed in the spinal canal is the spinal cord, the superhighway of nerve bundles that descend from the brain. A disc, between each of our vertebral bodies, cushions the fragile vertebra and allows motion when needed.

The discs are an engineering feat indeed. The outside, or annulus, is made of circumferential interwoven fibers, which interlock and attach to the vertebral bodies above and below. The inside of the discs are more gelatinous and, in concert with the annulus, are able to uniformly absorb and distribute pressure in a symmetrical pattern, so as not to destroy the structure's integrity. When the spine is stressed in any direction, the discs bear the brunt of load and redistribute it evenly. In severe cases of load and consequent asymmetry beyond the disc's mechanical strength, disc herniations or protrusions can occur.

Facet Joint Function

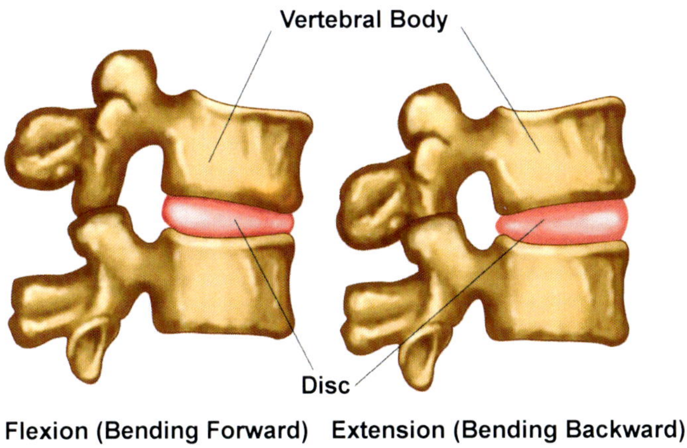

Facet joints are spinal joints where two vertebral bodies interconnect, yet they enable motion to proceed with ease. Each vertebra has two sets of facet joints, one right and left pair facing upward, and another right and left pair facing downward. These hinge-like facet joints, located at the back of the spine, link the vertebrae together while still allowing motion. Facet joints are also synovial joints. This means each joint is cartilaginous and surrounded by a capsule which produces a fluid to nourish and lubricate the joint. Therefore, the joint surfaces are designed to move or glide smoothly against each other. These joints allow flexion (bending forward), extension (bending backward), and twisting. Excessive vertebral body movements are prevented by the stability of the interlocking facet design, thereby preventing damage to nearby neurological structures.

Lumbar and Sacral Spine and Relationship to Nerve Roots

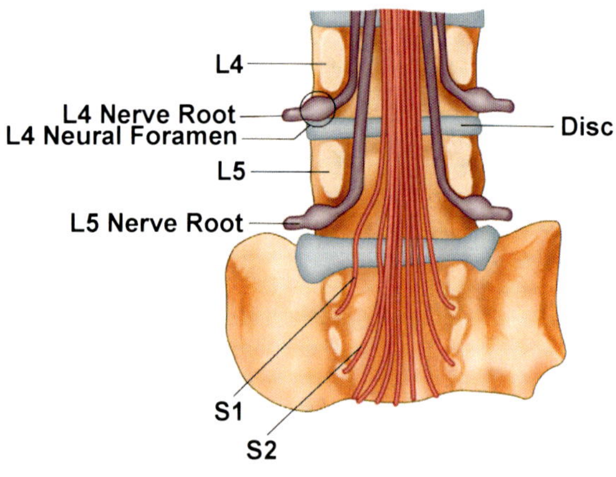

The neuroforamina, which are essentially holes located at each side of the spinal column in between each vertebral body, are where the nerve roots come out of the spinal canal and exit the safety of the bony spinal column on their way to the periphery. In this exit, they pass intimately by the discs and facet joints, hence any pathology in these structures, though minor, can affect the nerve roots. I view this as "zero lot line" property, where any infringement by one neighbor will cause chaos with the next.

CHAPTER 3

Common Pain Generators Originating in the Spine

There are many possible reasons for the spine to develop pain problems. As you are now aware, the spine is always involved in movement, and with movement, you may develop degenerative breakdown changes. Complicating the mechanical qualities, which can degenerate and become painful, is the nervous system that interweaves throughout the mechanical spinal structure. Even the slightest impingement upon these delicate nerves is capable of causing a massive pain response and disability, similar to how a minute grain of sand in the eye can bring you to your knees in tears. The point is - there does not need to be significant irritation or impingement upon a nerve for it to send pain signals that can be overwhelming. Spinal sources of pain are many and include nerve impingement, disc degeneration, spinal stenosis, facet pathology, spinal instability, post-surgical spine pain, nerve entrapments and vertebral body compression fractures.

Nerve root impingement, often spoken of as a "pinched nerve" is probably the most common pain complaint relating to the spine, and results in shooting pain down the extremity. This is called a "radiculopathy" from its Latin derivative, since the nerve root is involved. When occurring in the leg, it is also referred to as "sciatica". Radiculopathy and sciatica are merely descriptive terms; they fail to explain the reason for the pain, but only describe the pattern in which pain travels. This impingement occurs not peripherally, but usually in the spine, as the nerve roots exit.

Cross-section of Spine Showing Foraminal Disc Herniation

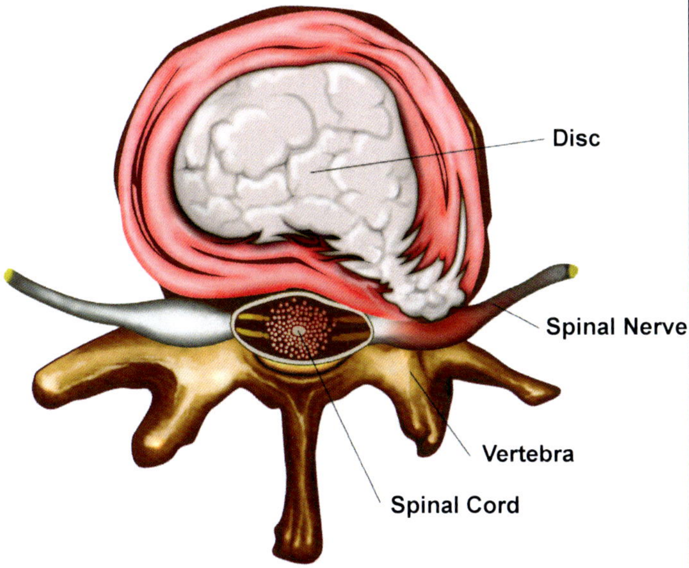

Common impingement reasons include nerves being caught between two vertebral bodies, nerves compressed by a disc herniation, or nerves trapped by large bony, arthritic osteophytic spurs. All of these processes can irritate or even render a nerve totally dysfunctional, if impingement is severe. In the younger patient, disc herniation is usually the culprit causing the pain. In the elderly, entrapment between vertebral bodies, as well as osteophytic arthritic compression - both mechanical degenerative processes, becomes more common. As the nerves course away from the spine, they can become irritated by nearby enlarged ligaments and muscles. This is commonly referred to as a peripherally "trapped" nerve which sometimes responds to surgical "release" or transposition to a less confined area. Nerves can also be the target of irritation derived from repetitive motions that interfere with proper nerve function.

Side View Cervical

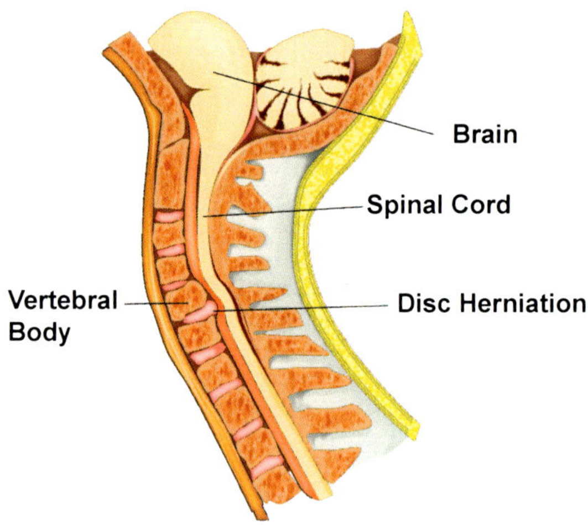

As a result of nerve root impingement, the patient may complain of numbness, tingling or weakness in various parts of the body. There may be localized pain in the back associated with the neurological complaints as well. Nerve root irritation in the neck or cervical spine area can cause symptoms in the neck, shoulders, arms, or hands. Nerve root irritation in the lumbar or low back area may cause back pain, numbness, tingling, and weakness in the legs and feet. A severe nerve root impingement in any area, where the entire spinal cord is being entrapped, may not only cause pain and numbness, but also difficulty walking, and possibly incontinence. This is a surgical emergency. Otherwise, impingement is rarely a surgical emergency if it involves only one extremity, even though there may be associated severe pain along with weakness and numbness. Though nerve root irritation often causes pain down an extremity, it may also only cause back pain with some associated muscle spasm, in the total absence of any other signs of neurological dysfunction.

Disc Herniation with Spinal Cord Compression

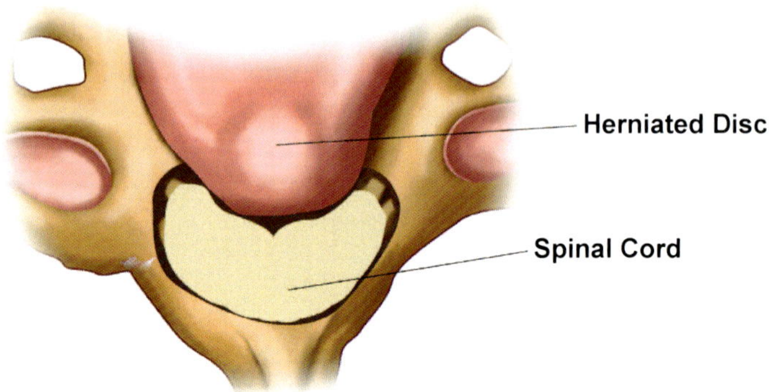

Discs do not need to touch nerve roots to be painful, as they can be inherently painful on their own. A large disc herniation, though often causing associated neurological irritation, may only disrupt some of the ligaments in the back, namely the posterior longitudinal ligament (PLL). This occurs most commonly when the disc protrudes straight backwards, and not in the more common slightly one-sided (posterolateral) direction. When the PLL is disrupted from its normal anchoring site to the bone, severe back pain can develop. Even if a surgeon were to remove the disc herniation, the remaining ligamentous injury would result in persistent back pain. Hence, the surgery would be a failure in terms of gaining pain relief from disc removal.

Not everyone with disc pathology has pain. The

majority of people over the age of 50 have some form of disc changes on an MRI, even though they may never have had back pain problems. Thus, it is important to obtain a very careful history and physical exam, to correlate the pain problems to any inciting events. Geriatric patients have copious disc and spinal pathology on MRI scans resulting in impingement, but this does not always correlate with pain. Paradoxically, they often are totally pain-free. The radiological findings are just incidental in these situations, having no clinical importance. A disc bulge, a small protrusion from its usual place between the vertebral bodies, causes no symptoms in most patients. However, if the spinal canal is small due to congenital or arthritic reasons, this seemingly inconsequential bulge can cause nerve root irritation that would not happen in the otherwise copious space in a healthier spine.

A disc protrusion and herniation is a more extreme form of a bulge, and more likely to cause symptoms. A disc extrusion is the most extreme form of a disc herniation, in which case the herniated part of the disc is actually totally separated from the remainder of the intact disc. All of these versions of disc pathology are casually referred to as "disc herniation", which can cause quite a bit of confusion amongst patients, as they claim their neighbor had a "disc herniation" that got better in 3 weeks, so why hasn't theirs? Well, as I explain to my patients, there are "disc herniations" and there are "disc herniations"; extreme variability in the level of pathology is inherent in that term.

Disc herniation pain is classically made worse with a "straight leg raise" maneuver. This is performed by laying a patient flat and raising the affected leg off the table. This maneuver actually lengthens the distance the nerve has to travel down the leg, which will exacerbate the pain if the nerve is already pinched. You can compare this to what happens when you pull back the string on a bow with an arrow; essentially the string (nerve) is a fixed length, so it pulls on the bow (disc) to which it is tethered.

Besides disc herniations, there can also be a disc annular tear, radial tear or radial fissure. A radial tear or fissure is any tearing that begins within the center of the disc and progresses like a spoke outwards to the annular level. There are different degrees or levels of annular tears, with a full thickness tear completely traveling through all the layers of the annulus. Disc degeneration is associated with radial and annular tears, often viewed as stemming from the natural aging process, though a history of trauma to that disc may have served as a catalyst to this degenerative process. It is important to understand that not all radial or annular tears are painful. They are found in asymptomatic patients, and it is poorly understood why some tears are extremely painful and while others are not. There is evidence that the small sensory and pain nerve fibers that normally surround the disc may make their way into the disc through these tears. As they pathologically grow into the disc where they don't belong, they may start to inappropriately send off painful signals. In a healthy disc, nerves do not grow into that area.

Examples of Disc Problems

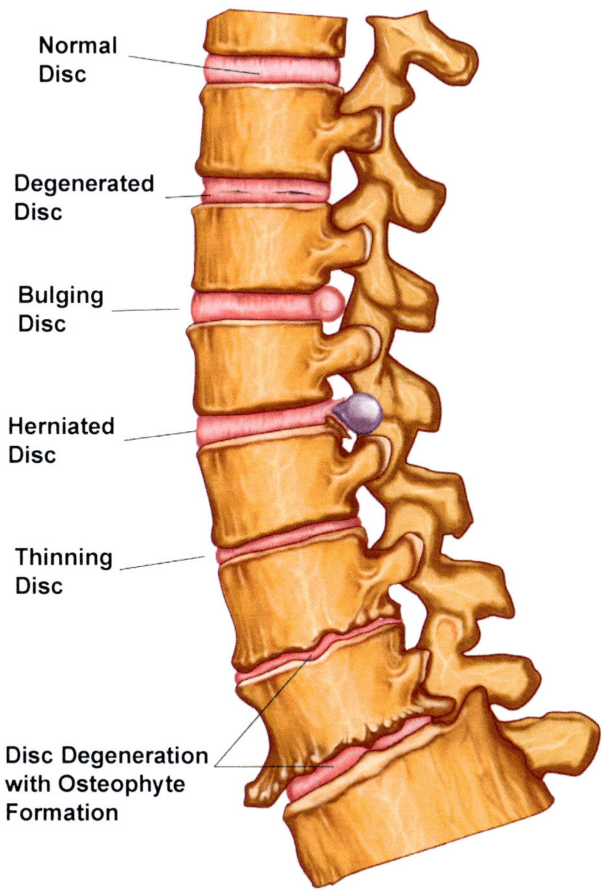

Yet another category of painful disc pathology is disc desiccation. As the name implies, the discs are usually lacking the normal hydration they require to maintain the cushioning effect, and for this reason, maintenance of distance between the adjoining vertebrae becomes a problem. Disc desiccation is usually a progressive process seen commonly in the elderly, and sometimes in the younger population, where it can be quite painfully symptomatic. The diagnosis is typically made from a review of the MRI scan showing a "darker" disc as compared to the others. A darker disc on the MRI scan is the result of a lack of water, or hydration. Accompanying this finding, there is often a narrower disc space, and possible signs of more aggressive disc degeneration.

As the disc space narrows, upper and lower aspects of vertebral bodies, referred to as "endplates," collide with each other. This "bone on bone" phenomenon is a significant pain generator. The end point of severe disc desiccation and degeneration is arthritic spurs, connecting the vertebral body from the one above to the one below. This is your body's way of minimizing motion at that disc space level, hence, minimizing pain. Remember, where there's no movement, there should be no pain. Eventually, that entire segment may "auto-fuse" one vertebral body to another, and the role of the disc will no longer be of relevance. These patients tend to complain of nonspecific aching diffuse low back pain, made worse with sitting.

Every vertebra in your spine is a miracle of construction; all the nerves go through small passages between the vertebrae, called "intervertebral foramen", to reach the organ or muscle they serve. Likewise, the bony spinal canal provides protection for the spinal cord, that frail ropey conglomerate of all the nerves, as the nerves exit the spine and travel down from the cervical area towards the sacrum. Spinal stenosis is probably the most common terminology used when referring to the elderly, degenerated spine. Spinal stenosis is a generalized term for bony overgrowth and ligamentous overgrowth, including calcification and disc degeneration, all of which can serve to result in the closing of the spinal canal or its associated neuroforamina. This degeneration and closure can be excruciatingly painful, and may result in weakness. It can occur at one level, or sometimes many levels. It can exist limited to the spinal canal, or limited only to the exiting neuroforamina at one level, bilaterally (right and left), or at many levels. Much like the terminology of "disc herniation," there are wide variations in what is collectively referred to as "spinal stenosis". Therefore, there are also variations in treatment responses.

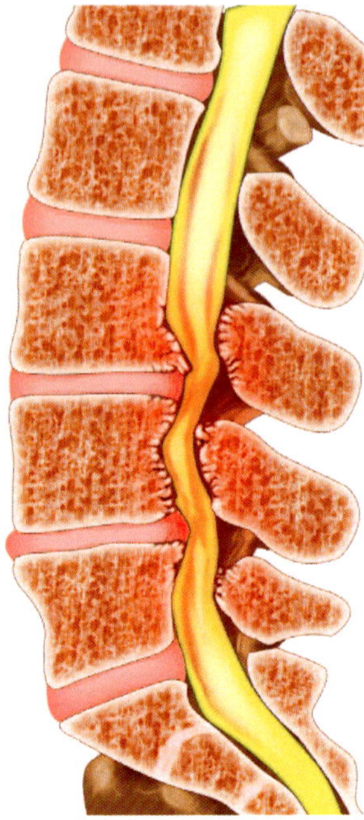

Spinal Stenosis

Spinal stenosis most commonly involves the lumbar spine, as this bears the brunt of the weight and motion. Less often, it involves the cervical spine, while thoracic spine involvement is a true rarity. In its most severe form, spinal stenosis can clamp down on the nerves causing persistent pain, or cause pain limited only to ambulation, referred to as "neurogenic claudication." These are the patients who prefer to walk hunched slightly forward over their walkers or shopping carts in the stores. This hunching or flexing forward of the spine, tends to open up the spinal canal and give them some relief. You will also see these patients in the mall, walking from one bench to another bench 20 yards away or so, before stopping and sitting. This way, they can regain the strength and sensation in their legs after the onset of neurogenic claudication. These patients will also be seen leaning forward over their shopping cart handles at the grocery store, effectively assuming a posture that maximally opens the spinal canal. This type of claudication differs from vascular claudication, as the former involves the legs diffusely and is relieved when sitting or leaning forward, while the latter is specific to a lack of circulation causing a muscle cramping or burning, often in the calves, relieved when walking is stopped, and is independent of change in posture.

Spinal stenosis can occur congenitally, from birth, associated with a smaller caliber spinal canal. In these cases, you will see symptoms often before age 50. This is quite rare, and references to spinal stenosis most often refer to the elderly with degenerative causes. Early onset of spinal stenosis must also be evaluated for rheumatologic diseases, such as ankylosing spondylitis. There are many rheumatological diseases which can prematurely cause spinal degeneration. Proper and early diagnosis with treatment, especially with the recent, very effective biological agents, will often avert the painful consequences seen in later courses of the disease.

Spondylolisthesis

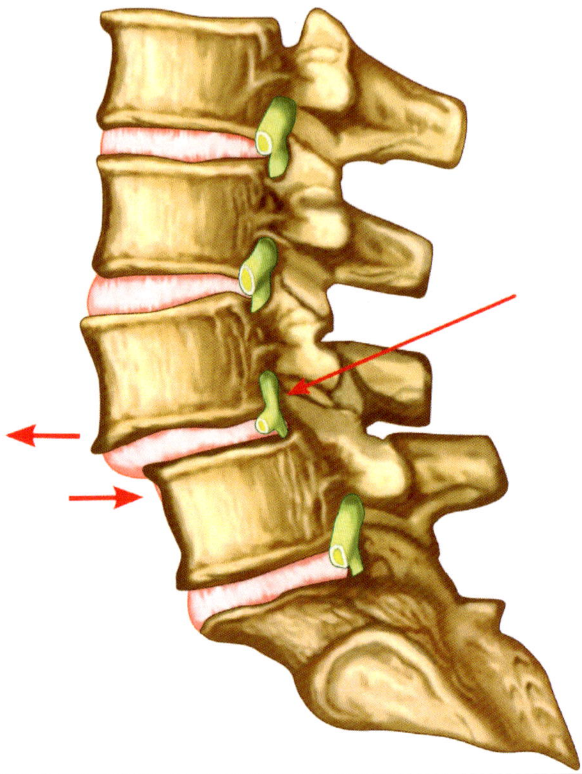

Spondylolisthesis refers to the forward slip of a vertebra over the one just below it. The different grades of slippage, from grade 1 to grade 4, have various degrees of associated pain producing expectations. Some people have no pain at all with this condition. For example, a grade 1 slip, which is less than 25% of movement of one vertebral body over the other, is often asymptomatic. However, a grade 4 slip, where there's essentially a complete disassociation of one vertebral body from the neighboring one, will result in severe pain and neurological deficits, including paralysis, as the spinal canal essentially gets obliterated. An ordinary x-ray can detect this condition, with dynamic motion detected on comparison of flexion film (leaning forward) and extension film (leaning backward). Compression of the nerves, and hence pain with neurological complaints becomes more evident with a more advanced "slip."

Low back and leg pain are common symptoms of degenerative spondylolisthesis. They are made worse with bending activities. There are several non-surgical treatments that have had success in holding pain at bay, such as exercise, braces, injections and medications. Very few patients require surgery, unless they are extremely, painfully symptomatic, in which case surgical fusion may be necessary. Sometimes spondylolisthesis doesn't even require treatment and will "auto-fuse" on its own, therefore guaranteeing no further slippage. If the vertebra isn't expected to slip more, the patient might just need to rest and to stop doing activities that cause pain.

Facet joints are another source of pain emanating from the spine. These joints occur on both sides of each vertebral body, right and left, as well as on both the upper and lower aspects of each body. They interconnect each vertebral body and aid in stabilization and alignment, reducing the risk of excessive motion. Facet joints, like any other joint in the body, are susceptible to injury and arthritis due to the constant motion they sustain. It is not unusual to see bony joint enlargement, arthritic bone spurs, or even cysts developing along the facet joints, especially when there is evidence of a slip or disc degeneration, which effectively causes this joint to approximate into a more narrow alignment. This facet degeneration is often referred to in the terminology of spondylosis. The joints contain a rich nerve supply; when the joint becomes inflamed or damaged, an aching and deep back pain is described. This pain is often made worse with extension, or bending backwards, which effectively brings the joint even closer together and exaggerates the arthritic compression.

I always ask my patients the open-ended question, “Where does it hurt?” With facet disease, the patients use their palm or entire hand, and rub it around their low back and gluteal area to describe facet-related symptoms. This is in direct opposition to the disc herniation or sciatica patients, who use one finger and point - very concisely - to the pattern of the pain. What they are essentially pointing at is the nerve’s path down the extremity. Facet pain rarely goes below the knee when involving the lower extremity, or the elbow when involving the upper extremity. It is not a sign of nerve compression; therefore, it never causes weakness or numbness. On the contrary, nerve-related pain that is due to compression from any source, tends to travel all the way down to the toes or fingers, and is quite often associated with neurological deficits.

Failed back surgery syndrome, also known as "post-laminectomy pain syndrome", is the unfortunate outcome of surgery which did not result in the anticipated goal of pain and symptom relief. Though a patient may have acute surgical pain, with healing for at least six months after major spine surgery, these failed surgical procedures result in patients who are still suffering for at least one year and longer after their operations. We all know of someone who has had many spine surgeries; sometimes with the same spine surgeon or sometimes each surgery with a different surgeon, in their desperate attempt to have a successful outcome. It is important to realize that this is not necessarily the fault of a poor surgical technique; it occurs in the best of hands and at the most prestigious institutions. It frustrates and angers the patient as well as the surgeon. No surgeon would agree to operate without a reasonable expectation of a positive outcome.

The possible reasons for this painful syndrome are many, but sometimes occur for no apparent reason. If the pre-operative status was that of severe nerve compression and injury, no matter what the source, then decompressing that area may not reverse the nerve damage that has already been done. Patients may develop scar tissue in the spine after surgery, which serves as a new source of pain.

Surgically removing that scar tissue would only lead to more scar tissue formation. Sometimes the pain is due to persistent muscle spasm from surgical dissection and trauma, or just a persistently painful scar from small, superficial, cutaneous nerve damage. Patients who are depressed and markedly deconditioned before surgery- a status not uncommon with patients with deteriorating spines - tend to have poorer outcomes.

As a general rule, patients who are poorer candidates for any spine surgery are those who have a history of obesity, smoking, advanced age, pain for longer than 6 months duration, psychological instability, are diabetic, deconditioned or had a previous failed back surgery. Patients with pain radiating down an extremity- radicular pain, do better than those with just pure neck or low back pain. Patients with secondary gain issues, such as desire for disability or extreme dissatisfaction with their careers, tend to have poorer outcomes. For the surgically-failed back patient, it is very important to undergo a comprehensive medical and radiologic workup to rule out reversible causes for their persistent pain. Often and unfortunately, the workup is normal, and technically the surgery was defined as a "success" by excellent anatomic results with radiological evaluation, but the procedure is considered to have "failed."

Compression fractures, common in the osteoporotic and elderly, can cause severe back pain. Compression fractures can also be seen with trauma or cancer, a disease for which the patient must be evaluated. A compression fracture is the collapse of a vertebral body due to one of the aforementioned conditions. The result is intense back pain which can last for weeks or months before slowly healing. Occasionally, though fortunately rarely, the bony compression affects the nerves or spinal canal, obviously making the situation worse. This condition is not a surgical emergency unless there are significant neurological deficits.

The unfortunate result of this type of fracture, besides pain, is that one fracture may have a domino effect, causing more fractures in the near future. This occurs because each fracture tilts the spine at a slightly unnatural angle, causing new and excessive stress on nearby vertebrae. Multiple compression fractures will cause your spine, and hence your posture to tilt forward (kyphosis), making ambulation more difficult. Reaching for things and looking straight ahead or upwards becomes quite arduous. As you bend forward even more, you can compress your lungs causing serious, if not fatal pulmonary complications. With heightened concern and screening for osteoporosis, this spinal complication is thankfully becoming less frequent.

CHAPTER 4

The Painful Truth about Back Pain

Though this book will cover all aspects of pain, the majority of the population's experience with discomfort is back pain. Back pain has taken center stage. I expect that back pain will remain a difficulty for the foreseeable future. There are some basic facts that everyone should familiarize themselves with about back pain. Too many patients feel their personal experience with back pain has not been recognized sufficiently, and perhaps this analysis will give them hope.

There are changes taking place all the time in the approach to, and the delivery of information to patients and caregivers. The advent of the computer and the Internet has inundated us with the latest information available, which, of course, empowers the patient. Hopefully, this will enable the suffering patient to avail himself or herself to superlative advice at the primary care level, rather than having to wait until advanced pain needs the attention of more specialized care.

An acute attack of back pain usually evokes the question, "Why did this happen?" The majority of acute back pain sufferers have no recollection as to what they did to cause their pain. They start self-evaluating whether they did anything unusual in their routines of work, driving, exercising, and taking care of the home and family. They all tend to blame it on things like lifting the groceries improperly, taking that extra long car ride, or sitting too long at the computer. But, don't we all do these things? Is this really the culprit? Yes, we all occasionally become "weekend warriors," physically exerting ourselves at projects or in the gym. However, that pain is to be expected, and is often referred to as a "good pain." Indeed, the majority of back pain seems to strike without any defining reason at all! Most often, it's noticed first thing in the morning as we begin to walk and stretch. Most of us ignore it, take a warm shower, and the pain experience is fleeting. However, there is a significant portion of the population who are less fortunate. That pain problem can linger with them throughout the day, become nagging, and compromise their ability to work or perform the activities of daily living.

A stunning 80% of the population experiences back trouble at some time in their lives, with many having back pain recurrences. Some survey results show that about 50% of the population had back pain during the prior year. Back pain is so common, it is often thought of as a part of the natural evolution of mankind, as we progressed from walking on all four extremities to walking upright. Some feel that the spine didn't evolve to support this change in posture as compared to the rest of the body. Back pain is common among all cultures with a peak incidence between the ages of 30 and 50, although 15% of adolescents will suffer from back pain in a milder form. People tend to assume if the back pain is agonizing then there must be something seriously wrong. In reality, far less than 1% of acute back pain episodes are associated with worrisome pathology or disease. The exceptions to these examples are the very young or the elderly, with both of these populations needing more aggressive medical evaluation for such acute episodes. It should be reassuring to know that there is an overwhelming incidence of minor pathology seen in acute back pain sufferers.

When it comes to the sexes, women complain of back pain more often than men. This may be for many reasons, including the wear and tear on the woman's body during pregnancy, childbirth, and child rearing, as these are physically taxing and can excessively strain the spine. Additionally, women are more prone to osteoporosis with age. Higher incidences of reported back pain in women may also be due to their greater willingness to seek medical care for pain-related issues as compared to their male counterparts. This is arguable, however, since men are often found to be less tolerant of pain.

It is logical to realize that our posture - how we sit and stand- can affect the incidence of back pain. Many of the back pain prevention groups and gurus focus solely on improving posture, both in sitting and standing positions. Posture, strength, and fitness programs are, therefore, very effective in preventing recurrences of back pain. They strengthen the body's core. Core strengthening simply means that all the muscles, both in the back and abdomen, are strengthened. The end result is that you become less reliant on the spine for support as the muscles can carry much of the weight and stress load. My analogy to this is the big red and white radio towers we often see as we travel down interstate highways. These towers are spindly structures, similar to a spine, and often ascend to 500 feet or more in elevation. I have yet to hear one of these towers getting structural damage or falling, even during tropical storms and hurricanes! Why is this true? It's not because of the innate strength of the tower, but due to the support of the guide wires. These wires come off every 100 feet or so, and minimize the shifts and bends the structure would otherwise experience during weather-related incidents. In this example, the guide wires are analogous to the muscles that support the "tower" or spine equivalent.

Bodily habits, lifestyle, and nutritional issues all affect the incidence of lower back pain. Obviously, the less active lifestyles tend towards less core support and a greater incidence of back pain. Therefore, obese patients often have more frequent complaints of back pain, due to their being deconditioned, as well as to the excessive weight load on the spine. When you realize that the lumbar spine has a width equal to that of your wrist, it becomes quite evident that, holding up your weight with a bony spinal structure that is wrist-wide is going to lead to trouble, especially for the morbidly obese and deconditioned individual. Often, the deconditioned, obese, young patient will be pain-free until his 50's, at which time his body can no longer compensate, and more aggressive, degenerative changes compound upon themselves. There is evidence that people on a poor diet, people with vascular disease, and people who smoke are more likely to have degenerative disc disease. This, in time, can translate into back pain. Even poor oral hygiene has a significant association with lower back pain!!!

Many people believe that, having an episode of back pain, or even having up to a year of significant, intermittent back discomfort, will disqualify them from their jobs or their ability to seek gainful employment. This is not true, as intermittent back problems are present even amongst the highest performing white collar executives and manual laborers. Having back pain is not a ticket to disability or early retirement. It is imperative to work around your pain and remain a productive member of society. When you are unhappy at work, the coexistent stress and depression are additive to your back pain symptoms. Therefore, it's important to vigorously engage in the challenges of work, as this mental and physical distraction has been shown to decrease one's inward focus on the self. As you engage in an outward career focus, the back symptoms seem to abate. I always tell patients that throwing themselves into their work, within reasonable limits, may paradoxically be the best cure for their back pain complaints.

It is an unfortunate market when people augment their pain complaints in a work-related injury or accident. These patients may then have an incentive to accentuate their complaints of pain and disability for financial gain and time off from work. This corner of the medical market unfortunately ties up the court system, results in higher insurance premiums for all of us, and may result in causing others to be unable to afford health insurance.

Though challenging, fortunately there are enough respected and qualified workers compensation and personal injury health care workers and physicians, who have the clinical acumen and skills to accurately evaluate these patients. These are performed with an accurate history and physical exam, close attention to the radiologic workup, and observing patients' body language, which may more accurately describe pain, as opposed to a verbal presentation alone. It is a humane system though, in our society, that workers sustaining major injuries and people who are unfortunately maimed in accidents, have leverage in the court system. They are entitled to reasonable financial reimbursement, and must not be turned away to suffer in their impaired state.

The flip side to this population is the athlete who has every incentive to get back to the game after an injury. These sports figures tend to deny or underestimate their injury in order to rapidly return to the sport they love so much, with the hefty financial rewards their performance allows. Unlike work-related injuries, the doctors are urging the professional athlete patients to take even more time off, thus allowing medical recuperation and minimizing risk of repeat injury.

Often when there is a back pain problem, people complain of a "weak back" or weakness in their extremities. It is entirely possible to have weakness with back pain, but most of the time no true weakness is found. This is an important differentiation to understand. What occurs with any pain condition is the production or augmentation of pain with physical exertion. In the fear of provoking their pain, patients will give suboptimal efforts on strength during physical examination. On the surface, this makes it appear as though they are weak. In reality, it's an avoidance technique that is normal and expected in human nature. It is not true weakness, but instead, a "voluntary guarding" or "give-way" weakness on exertion, which should be differentiated from true weakness on the medical records.

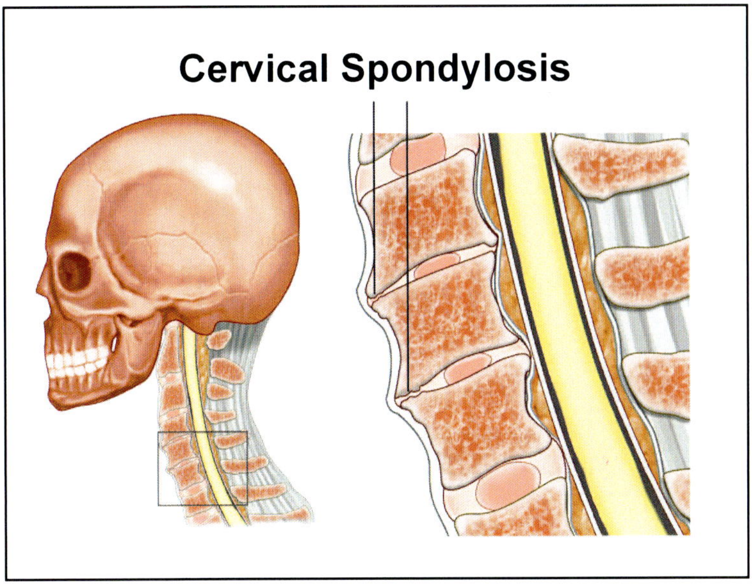

As we age, there is an accumulation of degenerative changes in the spine as a normal part of the aging process. These degenerative changes will be detailed in subsequent chapters, and include narrowing and degeneration of the discs, facet changes or spondylosis, and some spinal canal narrowing. These changes occur no matter how "good" or "bad" you have been to your back. You're not going to find a "normal" or "unremarkable" MRI scan on a geriatric aged person. The benefit of this knowledge is in knowing that your "margin of forgiveness" narrows, in terms of the spine, as you get older. In other words, the twisting, heaving, and lifting you may have tolerated without incident in younger years, may now have repercussions of pain. Therefore, proper knowledge of "body mechanics,"- or how to use your body mechanically most efficiently, without causing undue strain on the degenerative spine- becomes more important in the elderly. The development of acute back pain in the elderly, with associated multi-level, expected degenerative findings on an MRI scan, does not imply that something suddenly, anatomically went wrong and shifted. As a matter of fact, the MRI scan before the acute onset of pain would very likely look no different from the one taken when the geriatric patient is suffering. Pain relief in this patient population does not mean the MRI images became less pathological looking; indeed, there will be no change. As mentioned, the margin of error in moving the wrong way and causing back pain in the elderly is more minimal than in the younger adult.

Though the development of a degenerative spine may have some association with lifestyle, it can also have a genetic component. Collagen and protein strands, the materials that "bind" us together, may be inferior in some people, and passed down genetically. Those people at genetic risk should be especially diligent in maintaining proper diet, exercise, conditioning, and avoid cigarette smoking. These are the major lifestyle variables in the development of back pain. Though back pain may be a significant problem in the mid-life years, the severity tends to ebb in the later decades of life.

The responsible person, especially after suffering from one incident of back pain, will learn to be more vigilant concerning activities that can aggravate his propensity toward the recurrence of back pain. The activities that may increase the risk of provoking or worsening back pain, both lumbar and cervical, include lifting heavy weights suddenly, stooping and prolonged bending, twisting and repetitive reaching, excessive vibrations such as encountered with operating jackhammers, repetitive handling tasks, poor seating without back rest and arms supports, and improper heights of the components to computer workstations.

With awareness of these factors and good management, the future of the backache sufferer can look quite bright. There is rarely a reason to give up or change jobs and, in fact, maintaining gainful employment is most beneficial. The longer you are excused from work due to back pain issues, the less likely you are to return to work. There's an unfortunate, negligible return to work rate after six months of leave due to pain issues. It is therefore the goal of all physicians dealing with patients in pain to return them to work as soon as it is reasonably and safely possible, even if initially it's just for a few hours per day. The responsible patient will lose weight, undertake a rehabilitation and fitness program, and follow a home routine exercise program. Though there is no magic bullet, good common sense will help you alleviate most back pain dilemmas.

CHAPTER 5

Non-Spinal Conditions Causing Pain

There are many other causes of back pain other than those originating in the spine. Arthritis is one of the most common sources of non spinal-related pain. There are many types of arthritis, each with its own unique treatment options. Therefore, the sub-type of arthritis needs to be investigated. Arthritic inflammation can be confined to a small area of the body, such as within a single joint, or it may be widespread, such as in rheumatoid arthritis. Tissue irritation or damage also results in inflammation, resulting in swelling, redness, heat and loss of mobility. Inflammation of a joint is called arthritis. Inflammation of a tendon is called tendonitis. Certain types of inflammation can be chronic and persistent, perhaps because of repetitive movement irritating the joint. Sometimes it is because of immune reactions, infections, or deposits of abnormal materials, such as is found with gout. Bone and joint inflammation can be crippling, but immediate treatment can prevent permanent joint damage.

Osteoarthritis (OA) is the most common degenerative form of arthritis. It is caused by chronic joint wear and tear and is most commonly seen in people over the age of 55, obese patients, and those with a history of joint trauma. It most commonly involves the more distal joints in the fingers, but may also involve a single larger joint, or many large joints such as the hips and knees. Rest tends to make the pain from OA subside. The sound or sensation of "grinding" and "popping" as one degenerative joint surface rubs against another is very common. Rarely is there swelling or redness.

Osteoarthritis is in direct contrast to rheumatoid arthritis (RA), which is an autoimmune disorder. Therefore, RA may be associated with inflammation and destructive changes throughout the entire body. It typically involves women between 35-50 years old, but can strike at any age. Even the pediatric population can be affected, in comparison to OA, which affects the older population. As with many autoimmune disorders, we are always unsure as to why they are triggered in any individual. We consider heredity, viruses, and bacterial infections as all possibly being part of the process triggering the disorder.

"Joint arthritis" of non-spinal origin, usually located in the nearby hips and shoulders, can often clinically present with neck or low back pain with associated radicular radiating pain down to the extremities as though from a spinal source though there is no spine or nerve root impingement pathology. "Sometimes the best treatment for low back pain is a hip replacement" is a common saying amongst orthopedic surgeons. Patients of senior age who have "arthritis of the spine," i.e. spinal stenosis, also have arthritis in the major joints such as shoulder, elbow, hips and knee. These comorbid, arthritic conditions can radiate pain to localized areas, thereby mimicking spinal arthritis or spinal stenosis.

Every week I see patients who befuddle their orthopedic and spine surgeons regarding the source of their pain. For example, we often perform hip joint injections in someone suffering from lumbar spinal stenosis and hip degenerative changes. If the pain is completely relieved, then we can confirm the hip is the source of the pain instead of the spine, hence the patient would benefit from hip replacement surgery and not spine surgery. Needless to say, these differentiations are important to recognize.

Many conditions are referred to as fibromyalgia syndromes, which are a group of disorders characterized by achy pain and stiffness in soft tissues, including muscles, tendons and ligaments. The pain and stiffness may occur throughout the body or might be restricted to specific locations, as in the myofascial pain syndromes. Fibromyalgia throughout the body is more common in women than in men. Men are more likely to develop myofascial pain or fibromyalgia in a specific area, such as a shoulder, from muscle strain. Fibromyalgia isn't dangerous or life-threatening, but persistent symptoms can be very disruptive and wearing as the gnawing pain persists.

True fibromyalgia is pain that usually involves tender points, or "trigger points", in all four quadrants of the body. These quadrants include the upper left back and arm, upper right back and arm, lower left back and leg, and lower right back and leg. The patient usually also complains of accompanying irritable bowel symptoms, fatigue, sleep disturbance, and depression. The patient usually sees many physicians in his attempt to get adequate treatment and often, unfortunately, comes back empty-handed.

There is a belief that fibromyalgia involves an imbalance in neurotransmitters, serotonin and norepinephrine in the brain and brainstem. There are newer medication modalities targeting these pathways, often referred to as SSRI's (selective serotonin reuptake inhibitors). Many of these medications are similar to anti-depressants but are marketed for the treatment of fibromyalgia, rather than for the treatment of depression. Physical therapy, keeping active by "pushing through your pain," and psychiatric evaluation and treatment of the co-existent depression, are the mainstays of therapy. While sometimes limited, tender muscle or trigger point injections are helpful. It is important to evaluate the patient for underlying disorders such as nutritional and electrolyte imbalances, thyroid disease, and other hormonal or rheumatologic disorders.

The term "pain referral patterns" is important to understand after the discussion of joint pain and myofascial pain. It is important to be aware of which joints or muscle groups radiate to different parts of the body. Often, the pain complaint is the "smoke" and it's imperative to know where the "fire" exists, instead of only addressing the "smoke,"- such as giving pain medications when a joint is causing the severe pain. In this case, a simple joint injection may alleviate all of the discomfort.

A more common example of pain referral patterns is angina, or lack of blood flow to the heart. The patient with angina may complain only of shoulder or arm pain with associated tingling. He also may complain of jaw pain or upper back pain-not the typical chest pain that we tend to link with heart disease. The astute physician would take a careful history and physical exam, of course knowing the importance of rapidly ruling out life-threatening diseases before embarking on the more benign arthritic treatments.

The peripheral nervous system (PNS) includes all the nerves outside the central nervous system - the brain and spinal cord. The PNS encompasses the cranial nerves that connect the head, face, and eyes directly to the brain and all the nerves that connect the spinal cord to the rest of the body. There are 30 pairs of spinal nerves emerging from the spinal cord in constant communication with the brain. As the nerves exit the spinal cord, they interconnect through plexuses, or nerve bundles, in the neck, shoulder, and pelvis, then divide again before traveling outward to more distant parts of the body.

Peripheral nerves are actually bundles of nerve fibers that may contain only sensory fibers, motor fibers, or a mix of both. They range in size from a microscopic fraction of a hair width to quite large, the size of one's thumb. Larger fibers convey messages that activate muscles and are responsible for non-painful sensations, whereas the smaller sensory nerve fibers transmit sensations of pain and control the automatic, non-voluntary functions of the body such as heart rate, blood pressure and temperature control. These smaller "pain transmitting" fibers are, unfortunately, the most prone to damage due to their small size and peripheral, more physically exposed, location. Common diseases such as long-standing diabetes, nutritional problems, HIV disease, and toxic medications used for chemotherapy often result in a diffuse, small fiber "peripheral neuropathy". This is the sensation of pain and/or numbness often confined to the extremities. It usually follows the distribution of someone wearing a stocking on the feet, or gloves on the hands, and is referred to in such terms. Peripheral neuropathies, for the most part involve the extremities, and rarely the torso.

Another form of peripheral neuropathy can be caused by a viral infection in one or more discrete nerves such as an infection caused by the herpes virus, called herpes zoster, resulting in the chronic pain condition of shingles. Don't worry, this is in no way related to the sexually-transmitted herpes infection, and has no implications of sexual infidelity. This fact I had to explain, and re-explain to one 90-year-old couple to prevent their 70-year marriage from turning sour when the husband developed shingles on his chest wall. His wife, after pulling me aside privately, insisted she has lived a full life, avoiding sexually transmitted diseases such as herpes, and she will leave him if he's catching diseases that could possibly harm her now. Of course, this wasn't the case and they remained a happy couple. The treatment for these neuropathies often involves trials of topical agents to desensitize the skin, medication trials, and injections with possible spinal cord stimulation if the pain is not too widespread.

Infection is another source of concern when it comes to evaluating pain. Starting with the nervous system, the brain and spinal cord are highly resistant to infection due to a protective dura or "plastic wrap" type material covering the entire system. However, when infection occurs, the consequences are serious and life-threatening. For example, meningitis, an infection and inflammation of the covering of the spinal cord and brain, is usually caused by a bacterial or viral infection. Aseptic meningitis is an inflammation of the meninges that is usually caused by a virus or is an auto-immune reaction caused by chemicals injected into the spinal cord. Encephalitis is inflammation of the brain itself and also stems from similar causes. Bacteria and other infectious organisms can reach the brain or spine from distant sites. They can be carried by the bloodstream (hematogenous spread), or can be introduced from penetrating injury or surgery. Infection may also spread into the brain from adjoining structures, such as the surrounding sinuses.

Bacterial infections, in various parts of the body, can cause significant pain syndromes. An abscess is a localized bacterial infection that can form anywhere in the body, including the brain, spinal structures, joints, organs, or soft tissue. Recent treatment for common infections such as pneumonia or urinary tract infections, followed by development of a pain syndrome, is worrisome in that an infection may have seeded somewhere else in the body and is now causing pain. This is more common if the initial infection was severe, requiring hospitalization, and was associated with "bacteremia" or the finding of the infection also spreading into the blood stream as diagnosed by blood cultures. Joint infections usually are associated with a warm, red, and tender joint with limitations of movement. These can be diagnosed with a joint aspirate, and must be treated aggressively for fear of permanent joint scarring and damage resulting in loss of function. Osteomyelitis, or infection of bone, can also be very painful as the periosteum, or covering of the bone, has a multitude of nerve fibers attached to it that are capable of producing pain. A kidney infection, also known as pyelonephritis, can cause severe back pain. A urine culture can help confirm this diagnosis.

Tumors are masses of new, uncontrolled tissue growth - benign or malignant- which cause pain or neurological loss by expansion and compression of nearby tissue, nerves or bone structures. They are often associated with an inflammatory response. Tumors may cause pain in various areas of the body in which they are located. Tumors may not cause pain for a long time and not until they are quite large or, on the contrary, may cause pain when barely detectable, depending on the tumor's location. When involving the gastrointestinal system, they may cause pain due to bowel obstruction and are often associated with nausea, vomiting, or constipation. When involving the bones, they will cause localized pain due to periosteum inflammation, irritating the highly sensitive covering around the bone.

When a tumor involves the spine, the patient may present clinically similar to a disc herniation or spinal stenosis patient. It is important to look for a tumor in the radiologic workup, especially in the elderly. Tumors can either be primary (originating from the organ or structure itself) or secondary (metastatic spread of cancer that originated elsewhere in the body). When it comes to tumors involving the spine, the vast majority of these are metastatic, coming from elsewhere. Common sources of spread to the spine are from the lung, breast, prostate gland, kidney, thyroid and lymphoma. Any tumor involvement in the spine can cause pain, numbness, tingling and weakness. The tumor could also cause difficulty with urination, loss of bladder control, and/or constipation. In the physician's medical history, tips that a tumor may be present include patient complaints of recent significant weight loss, night sweats, or constant gnawing pain, even at rest.

Headaches (HA), one of the most common complaints for which people seek physicians, are a pain or discomfort in the head that can be well localized or general. There are many causes of headaches, including those originating from the head itself or those referred from the neck area, called cervicogenic headaches. Though most causes for a headache are benign, more serious pathology must always be excluded. Additionally, the complaint of "the worst headache of my life" must be evaluated urgently for a cerebral bleed. Other acute headache urgencies include poorly controlled hypertension, meningitis, stroke and tumor. In broad terms, headaches can be broken down into "primary" or "secondary" causes. Primary headaches have no discernable cause and can be further divided into cluster, tension, and migraine headaches. Secondary headaches are associated with pathology being either benign or malignant, diagnosed by MRI or CAT scan, neurological exam, blood work, and visual exam.

Cluster Headaches

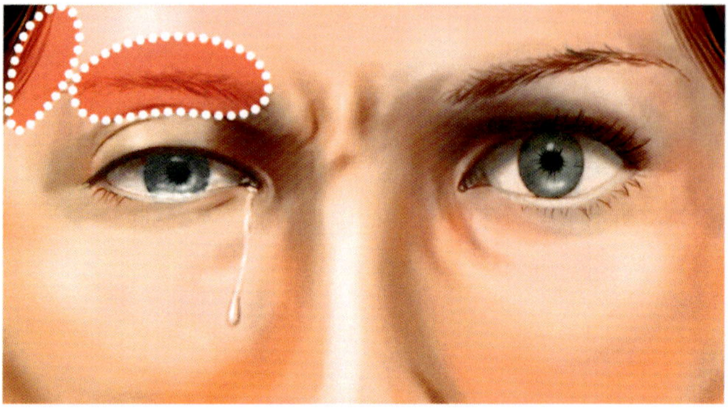

Cluster headaches may involve pain around one eye, along with drooping of the lid, tearing and congestion on the same side as the pain.

Starting with the first and most severe of the primary HA's, a cluster HA presents as severe unilateral pain behind the eye lasting from 20 minutes to 3 hours. Cluster HA involves mainly men in their mid-20s, and is associated with redness or tearing of the involved eye with nasal stuffiness. The cluster HA may recur several times a day, week, or month and always to that same part of the body, hence the name "cluster." Alcohol, vasodilating medications, and illicit drug use may play a role. The pain is so severe that these patients often pace and may actually bang their head against the wall or attempt suicide because the pain is so severe.

Tension Headache

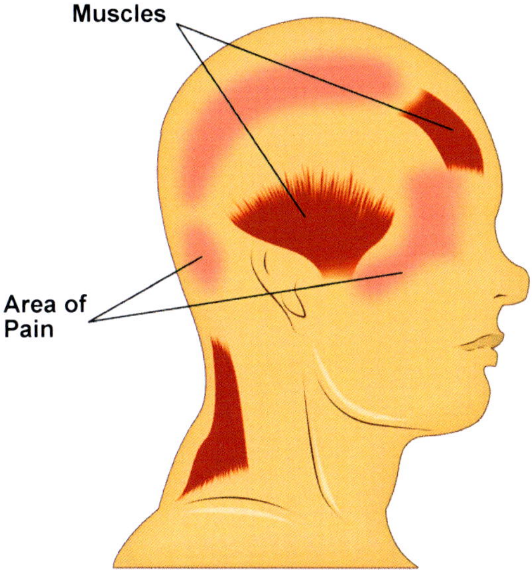

The second category of primary HA's - the tension HA – is the most common adult HA. The pain is described as a tight, band-like pain wrapped around the head as though wearing too tight a hat. This pain is triggered by stress, noise or bright lights, with predisposed patients having a history of sleep disturbance or depression. This HA may be associated with severe posterior neck muscle spasm.

The final category of primary headaches is migraines. Migraines affect all age groups but tend to be more common in women than in men. Migraines last longer than an hour but not more than a day, and may involve either both sides (bilateral) or just one side (unilateral) of the head. In some patients, there is an "aura" which forewarns the coming of the migraine. Auras may be variable, including numbness in the face, sensing particular smells, scintillating flashes of light, visual loss, unsteadiness in gait, or altered level of consciousness. Migraines are often associated with nausea and vomiting and may be triggered by certain foods, loud noises, bright lights, menses, depression, fatigue, or disturbance of the sleep-wake cycles such as with jet lag on long international flights. In contrast to cluster HA patients, who tend to pace around in the exam room, migraine patients will lay totally still in a darkened room with their eyes closed, avoiding all movements, loud noises, or any light.

Secondary headaches are caused by an underlying medical condition such as poorly controlled hypertension, infection, trauma, or space- occupying lesions. Typical space-occupying lesions of concern include tumors, bleeds or enlarging aneurysms. All secondary headaches require urgent, formal medical evaluation as they can be life threatening. The more ominous complaints associated with a secondary headache include "the worst headache of your life," abrupt headache onset, change in a usual headache pattern, or headaches in the age population less than 5 years old, or greater than 50 years old. Additionally, secondary headaches may be associated with physical exam abnormalities, seizures, syncope, exertion, sex or valsalva maneuvers (such as straining during a bowel movement).

There are many different types of pain which are associated with the aforementioned spine and non-spinal related origins. An understanding of the pain source and how it's transmitted will shed light on how to best approach the treatment. Some of the major types of pain include: nerve injury related pain, pain after surgery, visceral or internal organ pain, soft tissue muscular related pain, cancer pain and pain related to psychological disorders. These can all be confusing; however, in a broader and easier sense, pain can be divided into two broad categories: somatic and neuropathic pain.

Somatic pain is transmitted from small, pain-related "nociceptors" or nerve endings scattered throughout the body and designed to signal the brain when damage occurs to surrounding tissue. The classical example of this is pain from a scissor cut, a burn, or surgery. This is usually acute, well-localized discomfort, and responds well to narcotics and anti-inflammatories with expected rapid resolution. Seldom does this type of pain become chronic.

Somatic pain directly contrasts neuropathic pain which is from nerves not sending signals of damage to surrounding tissue, but damage to the nerves themselves! This pain is often described as more electrical, burning, shooting, and often less well localized. A common form of this is "funny bone" pain when you bang your elbow. Other, more chronic forms of this include sciatica-type pain from nerve impingement, peripheral neuropathy or shingles. The problem with neuropathic pain is that it tends to become more chronic and less responsive to medications. Narcotics often "blunt" the patient and make them indifferent to the pain, but the pain undoubtedly still exists. If there is a failure of initial conservative doses of narcotics and anti-inflammatories, often the next best medical treatment consists of anti-depressants and anti-seizure medications, due to the unique nerve pathways that neuropathic pain uses, differing from somatic pain pathways. Often times, repetitive nerve blocks help reduce the hyperactive state of these nerves, in a sense "resetting the fuse" of an overheated circuit. This is especially effective when treating acute pain. Also, by blocking these nerves, you are more likely to minimize the "spinal cord and brain imprinting" of this continuous, agonizing sensory input so that a cure can be more obtainable.

Psychogenic or psychologically-based pain is unique in the sense that, though the patient may be truly suffering, there is no discernable reason for the pain. This may be conscious, such as malingerers to avoid work duties. The more difficult cases are when it is subconscious or unconscious, such as a child developing leg pain with weakness to the point of falling down with vomiting when time to go to school due to some subconscious fears or believing dreaded experiences await there, whether real or perceived. This type of pain usually results in trips to many physicians with exhaustive testing all showing no pathology. Frequently, upon questioning, the patient is often indifferent to the fact that their leg occasionally experiences great pain or totally loses strength. One quick way to differentiate psychogenic pain in the leg, for example, as compared to neuropathic or somatic pain, is to do a nerve block in that limb making it totally insensate. If the pain still exists, most likely it's from a psychogenic source and further interventions are unwarranted.

CHAPTER 6

Initial Treatment before Seeking Professional Help

We all have occasional pain flares and illnesses for one reason or another- often never knowing the cause. Also, in every family there is a self-proclaimed "doctor" who is the first to give advice on treating an ailment due to "experience," whether true or not. This person ranges from the fascinations of the "shaman," in the more primitive Amazonian cultures (from which much of Western medicine is based) to the Jewish grandmothers (I had the greatest experience in my own family). The point is, for every undiagnosed ailment, there will always be many people giving free advice, labeling the diagnosis, and offering a home remedy treatment planned and laid out for you with their sincerity and best intentions in mind. In my home, growing up with physician parents, it was my grandmother who gave the strictest orders that everyone followed; and we thankfully always got better! In all deference to the grandmothers and shamans amongst us, there are some basic rules to follow when it comes to treating pain.

Although you may be suffering, remember the fact that the pain that comes on acutely (suddenly) also tends to go away acutely, often with no need for panic. However, the pain that comes on gradually, over months and years, is more difficult to treat. The treatments for these acute pain episodes are best managed by obviously stopping the activity causing the pain. Though this sounds like common sense, it's amazing how many weekend warrior types are undertaking landscaping renovations or moving furniture, only to develop back pain which subsides after 1-2 days, at which point they go back to the laborious project. In other words, if it hurts and you don't need to do it, then don't do it.

Rest and medications are the second line of therapy. Years ago, several days or weeks of bed rest was the treatment of choice for musculoskeletal pain disorders, especially back pain. The update on this is now no longer than one to two days, before slowly getting back to your routine. Why is there no longer prolonged bed rest? It was found that long term bed rest, especially in the elderly, was associated with rapid deconditioning of muscles, advanced osteoporosis, and a greater likelihood of getting complications such as pneumonia, hip fractures, and pulmonary emboli from deep venous thrombosis.

As for medications, there are many over-the-counter (OTC) medications to choose from, and it is the patient's preference as to which one to take. Keep in mind that aspirin is best kept to one daily, as larger doses are associated with a propensity to cause bleeding. Aspirin should also be avoided in the pediatric population as it is associated with Reyes Syndrome, a liver toxicity reaction. Acetaminophen (Tylenol) is not associated with bleeding and only lasts a few hours, so should be taken in that interval. It is great for reducing fevers and stopping pain, but does not have anti-inflammatory properties. Taking doses of 4000 mgs or greater of acetaminophen is considered dangerous and could cause liver damage. Some recent evidence suggests that maybe half of that dose is safely allowed. Acetaminophen is also in Tylenol #3, Percocet, and many other analgesics, so use caution to include all sources of this medication when evaluating your true intake of acetaminophen.

The non-steroidal anti-inflammatories (NSAIDS) are a large group of medications, which include generic names like Ibuprofen and Naprosyn, which equate to name brands such as Motrin, Aleve, and Advil, to name a few. These all last 4 to 6 hours per tablet, unless otherwise specified, and therefore should be limited to no more than a few daily. Similar to aspirin, they may be associated with bleeding for those prone to such a disorder. Therefore, they should be avoided in people with stomach ulcers and known bleeding disorders. NSAIDS are great for reducing inflammation, and consequently reducing pain, unlike acetaminophen which only reduces pain.

All of these oral agents bind to proteins in your bloodstream, which may in turn, displace other medications bound to these very same proteins. This is a more critical issue in people taking medications that require tight titration in order to maintain a very defined blood level, such as those on the blood thinner Coumadin, or on antiepileptic medication such as Tegretol. Consulting your doctor is always the best idea if there is any doubt.

Some of the OTC medications are topical and very effective, applied by rubbing onto your skin over the area of pain. This is the safest of all medication uses, since only negligible amounts get into the bloodstream. These topical OTC medications exist in abundance and, for the most part, are safe when used appropriately for a few days to treat acute pain episodes.

The vast majority of acute pain episodes are benign, will go away quickly, and have no associated significant pathology. However, there are always rare conditions that are the exception, or when taking OTC medications may be masking something needing closer professional medical evaluation. What are these warning signs suggesting the need for a more urgent physician's guidance? There are several scenarios requiring greater caution. Pain associated with fevers is always worrisome for infection needing culture and targeted antibiotic therapy, if appropriate. Weight loss, especially with night sweats, can be an early sign of a malignancy. Patients with a history of cancer and now suffering from pain should also be evaluated for a recurrence of cancer or metastatic disease. Coexistent sleep disturbance usually implies a more significant pain problem, especially if the OTC medications fail to give enough pain relief to allow a comfortable night's rest. Loss of neurological function is always a warning sign of significant nerve impingement. When this involves instability of gait and associated loss of bowel and bladder control, it is a surgical emergency. Prolonged, severe compression of nerves can lead to permanent nerve injury, even though the nerves were surgically decompressed. Lastly, those at extremes of age - the very young or aged - should seek medical guidance more urgently. Discussion of the aforementioned medications and acute pain guidance provides a very general outline; it does not apply to all patients. It is always important to initially consult with your physician if there are any doubts or coexistent medical issues.

CHAPTER 7

Physical Therapy

Physical therapy is one of the most common and accepted modalities prescribed for patients in an attempt to address pain issues, especially if associated with musculoskeletal derangements and loss of function. Inflammation and pain can be reduced with the help of a physical therapy program, including the low back pain that affects up to 80 percent of Americans during their lifetime. Physical therapy is the mainstay for initial treatment for any musculoskeletal condition, and has evolved into a formal and precise science. A physical therapy program is only as good as the therapist directing it, a fact known and appreciated by most pain physicians, orthopedic surgeons and spine surgeons. The physical therapist is often the "right hand" person for these physicians, and the therapist's skills help augment the surgical and interventional treatments, thereby giving the patient the maximum benefit. Quite often, with excellent physical therapy, there will be no need for the patient to undergo pain management procedures, surgery, or further medical management. Therefore, due to its safety and effectiveness, physical therapy is my first step in the pain recovery program.

Physical therapists are highly trained medical

professionals who require a graduate degree from an accredited physical therapy program and take a national licensure examination before starting to practice. They also require individual state licensure. Physical therapists are key members of the pain management community and independently take a history, perform a physical, and come to a diagnosis and treatment plan, which augments the physician's.

Because physical therapists receive specialized training in a variety of sciences such as physics, anatomy, and kinesiology (human movement), to name a few, they understand the mechanics of the body and how to get it moving efficiently again. A physical therapist will act as your coach, discussing with you the science of your body, its structure, and various modalities to improve and manage your musculoskeletal health condition, thereby lessening the risk of further deterioration. After examining you, the physical therapist will develop a unique plan individualized to meet your own needs, in order to most effectively restore function. There is a wide array of illnesses with musculoskeletal issues. A therapist can greatly assist in the recovery of such illnesses. These conditions range from back and neck arthritis, poor posture, repetitive stress injury, diabetic neuropathy, stroke recovery, and recovery from surgery or trauma.

When you see a physical therapist, you can expect a review of your medical history and a medical examination, including testing of strength, range of motion, coordination, balance, posture, and motor function. He will ask about your expectations and get a sense of your ability to rise to the challenge in order to meet your goals. Therefore, his role also has psychiatric overtones, as he learns what really motivates you while assisting you in harvesting your energy in the most productive way. The therapist will facilitate your integration back into the community with the pursuit of gainful employment, using new musculoskeletal skill sets if needed. Therefore, therapists tend to be very compassionate and empathetic people, listening to your needs and adjusting accordingly. The changes that are made are never tremendous or made overnight, but are slow and steady. These changes require a patient's continuous effort, and the therapist's encouragement towards realistic goals and expectations.

When treating the spine, there are two primary categories of physical therapy used: passive physical therapy and active physical therapy. Passive physical therapy focuses on decreasing pain by using modalities and manual therapy techniques. Emphasis is placed on the reduction of stress and tension on the musculoskeletal system by creating a relaxed environment while implementing physiologically correcting treatments. These treatments are considered to be passive therapies because they are done to the patient. Heat and ice are easily available and are the most commonly used modalities. Generally, heat is used for tight muscles and stiffness, while ice is most effective in reducing active inflammation accompanying acute injuries. In rehabilitation, heat is usually used to start a treatment in order to prepare the desired area for intense exercise, and ice is used to end a session in order to reduce any post exercise soreness or swelling. Electric stimulation such as Interferential Transcutaneous Electric Nerve Stimulation (TENS), High Volt Galvanic Stimulation (HVGS), and Microcurrent, are used for their specific physiological responses. In general, they modulate pain, relax muscle spasms, and create a pumping action in muscle groups to clear away waste products at a cellular level. When electrical stimulation is utilized with specific combinations of wavelength, frequency, and intensity, they can be very effective in treating spine conditions. Ultrasound is a common modality as well. It acts as a deep form of heat in which sound waves penetrate the skin, causing soft tissue to vibrate and create heat. In turn, the heat induces vasodilatation (increased blood flow) and promotes the delivery of oxygen and nutrients while removing cellular waste. Ultrasound is especially useful in relieving acute pain, reducing muscle spasms, and accelerating tissue healing. A combination of ultrasound and HVGS, called "COMBO", can be very effective in reducing localized muscle spasms and trigger points, commonly referred to as "pain generators." Another very effective passive therapy is called Iontophoresis. Lontophoresis is a method in which medication is delivered through the skin by the use of electric stimulation. For example, Dexamethasone is applied to the skin via an electrode under the negative pole, and the electric current applied repels the (-) ion while forcing the drug under the skin. The steroid then produces a localized anti-inflammatory response in the target area. It is very effective in the treatment of bursitis, tendonitis and acute inflammatory conditions.

Manual therapy is another type of passive physical therapy. It can be delivered in the form of joint mobilization. This uses techniques that address dysfunctional vertebral segments that interfere with normal activity or motion. Soft tissue mobilization treats muscles by restoring their normal resting tension. Finally, myofascial release is a method in which the body's connective tissue can be manipulated so that movement patterns are not restricted by tight fascia. Qualified manual therapists or "hands-on" therapists who have the proper experience best perform manual therapy that is goal-directed and tissue-specific.

Active physical therapy consists of prescribed exercises and manual techniques that are necessary to effectively rehabilitate the spine. Emphasis is placed on patient involvement and the goal of returning to pre-injury levels of function. The purpose of the exercises in physical therapy is to eliminate pain and to restore normal function wherever possible. When you are exercising for pain relief, as most patients are, you "move to the edge of the pain" or just into it, and then release the pressure and return to the starting position, to resume again when the muscles have eased. Activity-specific exercises are performed to simulate a patient's daily required activities. Physical therapy that safely mobilizes the spine and the surrounding tissue can help alleviate the pain and can have long-lasting effects. Stretching exercises can benefit everyone, especially patients with back and neck pain. The hamstrings, hip flexors, and hip rotators all play a key role in low back pain. Likewise, upper traps, scalenes, and other cervical musculature significantly impact the mechanics of the neck. If any or all are tight, it can result in severe pain and difficulty performing activities of daily living. For example, significantly tight hamstrings can cause a posterior pelvic tilt, resulting in a decreased lumbar lordosis. This can cause mechanical problems of the spine, difficulty with movement, and even cause injury when performing normal activities.

Targeted strengthening exercises also play a very important role in the treatment of spine pathology. More specifically, dynamic lumbar stabilization exercises are exercises designed to help keep the back strong and well positioned by targeting core muscles. It is very important that they are progressed correctly and that the appropriate technique is used. Early abdominal and back extensor recruitment with the spine supported in neutral is vital. Patients are then asked to maintain a "neutral spine" position while performing exercises of greater intensity, greater ranges, and with less support. This renewed positional awareness of the spine and the ability to recruit the proper muscle groups is the cornerstone of spinal stabilization exercises. Once the area is re-educated, most high-level activities can be performed with the confidence that the spine has the strength, endurance, and flexibility to handle the activity.

Although commonly overlooked, aerobic conditioning also plays a very important role in the treatment of musculoskeletal conditions. With greater cardiovascular fitness comes overall improvement in health and endurance. Many injuries occur as a result of overall fatigue and poor endurance. This results in the breakdown of proper posture or lifting techniques. Walking is therefore, generally very beneficial to all patients with chronic or acute pain. Walking 2-3 miles, three times per week is known to be very helpful. When walking is painful, using a stationary bicycle or an upper body ergometer can be a safe effective alternative. It is believed that 30-40 minutes of aerobic exercise has an added benefit of increasing the production of endorphins to control pain.

Today, pain relief exercises are commonly performed in the treatment of spine conditions. One of the most common approaches for back pain, especially if associated with disc problems, is the McKenzie Method, which is derived from a book by Robin McKenzie, a world-renowned physical therapist, titled Seven Steps to a Pain-Free Life. His method is hailed in many countries as the ultimate cure for back and neck pain using non-interventional approaches. The book recounts how he stumbled upon the pain relief that can be achieved when putting the pain-stressed body in a position of extension. This position of the body, in some cases, immediately relieved the pain. This was first noticed quite by accident when a patient was told to lie down on the exam table and await the therapist. The table was angled in such a way that when the patient was lying face down, his back was arched backwards at about 45 degrees, as this was how the table was positioned after the prior patient was examined while laying on his back (more like a beach chair position). When Dr. McKenzie came into the room and saw the patient in such a seemingly awkward position, he apologized profusely. The patient would not accept any apologies since he claimed that, in the arched backward position, he experienced greater pain relief than with any other modality in the past several months!

After examining the spinal anatomy more carefully in this position, Dr. Robin McKenzie began his series of innovative procedures for relieving specific types of back pain. Opening up the spinal column by stretching the back in the opposite or arched position, the pressure was released on the nerves and the patients had resolution of their previous leg pain. When this was done in a routine, slow and guided manner, patients often did not need their scheduled surgery. The McKenzie back and neck exercise program consists of seven separate exercises, using both extension (bending backwards) and flexion (bending forwards) techniques. Most patients have no need to use more than two of these exercises. Therefore, this is an easy technique that is not time consuming. By "centralizing" the pain, i.e. bringing it from the legs to the back, it becomes easier to treat and better is tolerated by the suffering patient.

Since ancient times, water has been used for its healing properties. Pursuing an aquatic exercise program, guided by a physical therapist, can be very rewarding in terms of pain relief and recovery from injury. Water walking, swimming, and flexibility exercises can help avoid surgery or other expensive invasive procedures. Aquatic therapy exercise reduces gravitational forces on the entire body while diminishing joint compression. Aquatics allows for greater comfort and ease of movement for patients, especially when land-based exercises increase pain. The surrounding water pressure and temperature assists in reducing inflammation and provides sensory input for postural awareness. The ideal pool would be heated and convenient, such as in one's backyard or apartment complex, so that the pool can be used frequently and conveniently to maximize program compliance. The aquatic activities discussed below should be performed at least five days per week, for 30 minutes or longer.

Though pain relief from aquatics does not come immediately, most sufferers find remarkable relief after two weeks of daily aquatics and often wonder, "Why didn't I try this earlier?" By being buoyant in a pool, with water reaching the level of the upper chest, the patient is effectively taking as much as 50% of the weight off the spine. Another way to achieve this is by hanging on a Styrofoam "noodle" or hanging on the side of the pool with the legs dangling below. The muscular heaviness of the lower body pulls down, while the buoyancy of the lungs pulls up. This combination helps distract or separate those disc spaces chronically being compressed by the effects of gravity. Essentially, it can function very much like traction, but it is a lot more enjoyable when done in the pool.

Corrections to bad posture are another way you can get relief of chronic pain due to mechanical or structural imbalances. If the sufferer wants a greater "cardio" workout, she can start slowly and gradually working up to water walking as rapidly as possible for a measured half-mile at least three times a week. There will be a significant lessening of pain for this patient in a very short length of time. The resistance of the water against the striding of the legs and the pushing of the arms against the water at the same time, both strengthens the muscles of the back and eases the muscle spasms caused by habitually bad sitting or standing postures. Eventually, the breaststroke or the Australian crawl can be utilized for muscle strength and toning, in addition to the aforementioned aquatic activities. Many of my patients enjoy it, feel well, and likewise enjoy the new social climate of which they have become a part.

Be conscious of the vertebrae and the discs between them, hold the shoulders back and tuck in the chin, while never hunching over, this will give maximum pain relief, when sustained over time. As with all things, making small but consistent adjustments to posture, body mechanics, positioning and self-care habits can add up to significant relief from debilitating pain. Good postural habits should be followed for the rest of your life to prevent any recurrence of the spasms that inhibit movement.

As evidence-based care gets greater attention in today's healthcare environment, physical therapists are treating muscular and skeletal disorders in a more integrated way. Studies have shown significant benefit from physical therapy in decreasing pain and gaining function. Furthermore, it may avoid the hefty expenses of medications, procedures, or surgery. Physical therapists have an assortment of techniques and tools which can be tailored uniquely to the individual patient. Effective treatment will focus on patient pain complaints, movement dysfunctions, mechanical and muscular imbalances, and educating the patient to minimize the risk of injury recurrence, thereby preventing pain from becoming chronic. It is clear that physical therapists are becoming an asset to physicians by assisting in the monitoring of patients, and by communicating and evaluating these findings and the patient's response to treatment. In the end, it is the multidisciplinary team approach that is most effective in treating all patients.

CHAPTER 8

Medications

Analgesics - medications which are used to treat pain- come in many varieties. They function by having effects on the nervous system via a complex system of various neurotransmitter pain pathways, both excitatory and inhibitory in nature. Most often, the medications target and mute the ascending input from the periphery to the brain, but in other instances, they may excite the descending neuro-inhibitory pathways which serve to reduce input into the spinal cord or brain. A common example of this is Ritalin, widely used as a stimulant. However, it causes excitation of inhibitory neurons in people with attention deficit disorder, thereby actually calming them down.

There are two broad varieties of analgesics: those that are over-the-counter (OTC) and others that are limited to prescription only. OTC medications are usually for mild to moderate pain and consist mostly of Aspirin, Tylenol, (acetaminophen) and non-steroidal anti-inflammatories (NSAIDs). The prescription medications require a physician's authorization. They are stronger, tend to have more side effects, and can be habit-forming in comparison to the relatively benign OTC variety. Prescription analgesics are reserved for moderate to severe pain and are most classically represented by opioids.

Acetaminophen (Tylenol) is probably the most commonly used OTC medication and is remarkably safe. It is used most frequently for pain and fever control. Though it functions as an analgesic and antipyretic, it has no true anti-inflammatory effects like the non-steroidal anti-inflammatories (NSAIDs) do. The main concern for long-term use of acetaminophen is liver toxicity, especially in doses approaching 4 grams or more per day. Recent recommendations are to allow no more than 2 grams daily. Acetaminophen is often combined with narcotics such as Percocet (acetaminophen and oxycodone). This fact is frequently overlooked when calculating acetaminophen exposure for patients taking a few additional pain medications.

Aspirin and NSAIDs are also available OTC, but in the higher doses, require a prescription. They include such common names as Naproxen (Aleve) and Ibuprofen (Motrin, Advil), and all work by blocking the formation of prostaglandins, a hormonal substance that plays a role in inflammation and its associated pain. Though these agents are potent anti-inflammatories, through the same mechanism of action they can also cause kidney toxicity, fluid retention, and bleeding stomach ulcers. Therefore, NSAIDs are used with more caution than acetaminophen for acute pain episodes with treatment lasting one to two weeks. At times, NSAIDs are used for months or years, in which case closer medical monitoring or use of a special "Cox II" category is employed. NSAIDs are commonly used to treat the pain of headaches, muscle aches, dental pain, menstrual cramps, arthritis, or athletic injuries. Some NSAIDs are also used to reduce fever in addition to acetaminophen. The size of the dosage is based on the type and level of pain, as well as the response to therapy. If stomach upset is present before or during the taking of this medication, the patient should take it with food. In certain conditions, such as medication for arthritis, it could take as long as two weeks before the full effect of the drug taken is felt, even when taken regularly. Possible side effects of aspirin, acetaminophen, and NSAIDs that require physician notification are upset stomach, nausea, vomiting, heartburn, headache, diarrhea, constipation, drowsiness, deafness, rash, and unusual fatigue. Rare allergic reactions such as rashes, itching, swelling, dizziness, and breathing difficulties do occur, so it's wise to be aware of the possibility and be alert to any of the adverse symptoms.

In addition to the NSAIDs previously described, there is the more unique, cycloocygenease-2, or "COX II" inhibitors, such as celecoxib (Celebrex). These are equally as effective as other NSAIDs, but are more selective in their blocking of cyclooxygenase, therefore minimizing the risk of bleeding, stomach ulcers, and kidney complications. Though they are more expensive than other NSAIDs, they are medically necessary and indicated in higher risk patients. Other COX II inhibitors have been removed from the market due to cardiovascular side-effects, but celecoxib has been extensively studied and is safe for long-term use.

Muscle relaxants are prescription medications that help relieve the discomfort from muscle spasm. There are many forms of muscle relaxants- some of the more recent ones are long acting, requiring only one dose per day. The reason these medications work is varied, but all decrease excitation of the nervous system, thereby causing sedation, which is the most common side effect. Some patients find this very helpful, while others find them so sedating that usage is only limited to "qhs," or, prior to bedtime at night.

Anti-depressants, not used primarily for depression in the pain management scenario, come in two main forms - the tricyclic and the serotonin blocking types. The latter increases the central nervous system's serotonin level, causing a suppression of pain signals. They both may have the additional benefits of improving mood, decreasing anxiety, and assisting in sleep, all of which can be associated complaints in the chronic pain patient. There is no addiction or abuse profile with any of these agents. To minimize risk of side effects, they are usually started at a low dose and slowly escalated to a more therapeutic, effective dose over weeks to months.

Tricyclics, especially amitriptyline, are used in pain conditions involving nerve damage, fibromyalgia, or headaches, especially when associated with sleep disturbance. Tricyclics have been used for at least a few decades and found to be very effective and safe. The prescribed dose is far less than one would use for true depression. The benefit of assisting in sleep occurs immediately, though the pain relief effect may take at least several weeks to be realized. Unfortunately, side-effects commonly occur, and consist of a "morning hangover" of excessive fatigue, dry mouth, constipation, urinary retention, and some dizziness upon standing first thing in the morning. These side effects, when mild, tend to minimize after several days. Tricyclics are avoided in the more elderly and frail, especially in a cardiac patient due to possible effects on the heart's conductivity. Unfortunately, often times the tricyclics with the most side effects are also potentially the most effective, and hence a double-edged sword in its usage.

More recently on the market, the selective serotonin (and norepinephrine) reuptake inhibitors SSRIs and SNRIs are anti-depressant agents and are also capable of offering pain relief. Similar to their tricyclic counterparts, they are effective for pain due to nerve injury, as well as fibromyalgia complaints. Some of the medications in this group work better for depression, while others are approved for pain control, such as duloxetine (Cymbalta). As a group, they are much better tolerated than the tricyclics but, unfortunately, not always as effective. I find it challenging to convince the patient to try one of the anti-depressants. They are convinced that I think they're depressed when that's not the reason for my prescribing them! However, I explain that I do believe by conquering the coexistent sleep disturbance caused by the pain, either by the use of antidepressants or muscle relaxants, the patient will be happier and more able to cope with his remaining painful malady.

Another category of prescription medications is the anti-seizure variety, or anticonvulsants. Though originally designed for the treatment of seizure disorders, many of these medications have subsequently been found to be very effective in treating painful conditions, especially that of neuropathic or "nerve damage" pain. Gabapentin (Neurontin) is a new generation agent typical for this group, which is now more commonly used than the older generation medications, typified by carbamazepine (Tegretol). They work by decreasing the firing rate of small pain fibers, similar to how they decrease the firing of nerves involved in seizure disorders in the brain. The newer anti-seizure medications seem to be much more effective than the older agents. Additionally, the new agents have much fewer side effects and a lower toxicity profile. There is virtually no need to check routine blood work, as was necessary with older agents such as carbamazepine. Additionally, the newer agents tend to cause fewer interactions with other medications the patient may be taking; therefore they are "cleaner" medications to use, especially by the more elderly, frail patient.

Opiate drugs are, by far, the most controversial of all prescription pain medications. They come in all varieties: short acting, long acting, oral, transdermal (transcutaneous), intranasal, intravenous, and even injectable into the spinal canal! They all work by stimulating certain pain receptors located naturally in your body, called "mu receptors". By stimulating this receptor, not only do they block pain transmission, but they also create a sense of euphoria, and hence, have a highly addictive potential. This feeling is similar to the "runners' high" that athletes often achieve after undergoing vigorous physical activity, followed by the release of the body's own natural endorphins, or opiates! If opiates are put in the wrong hands, such as those with addictive personalities, they more readily can become problematic, and abuse is more likely to occur. Therefore, the addictive personality patient types such as chronic smokers, drinkers, and gamblers have a higher risk profile for using such medication.

All opiates can be sedating, and may cause the side effects of confusion, constipation, or stomach upset. It's difficult to predict which patient will tolerate these medications and so it is always important to start with short-acting, low dose versions and increase as tolerated and appropriate. Your body will develop a tolerance to these side effects and, with time, a total resolution of side effects may occur. If the side effects are extreme, then no reasonable tolerance can be expected and the opiate should be discontinued.

The proper dosing of opiates is the key to their success. If you are finding yourself needing an opiate approximately four times daily, then it's best to schedule a routine dosing every 6 hours instead of waiting for the onset of pain. Regular dosing is the best way to maintain an appropriate drug level, and actually may result in less pain with less opiate use as compared to dosing only "as needed." Chronic opiate users are often put on a once or twice a day amount of slow release narcotic to aid in maintaining steady blood levels with occasional short acting analgesics given every few hours as needed. If the short acting or "breakthrough" medication is needed often enough, due to worsening pain or the development of drug tolerance, then the dose of the long acting opiate should be increased. On the other hand, if opiates are rarely needed and only used for more painful exertions or activity such as square dancing, then taking 30 minutes or so in advance to allow digestion and entrance into the bloodstream is best. I describe this as "anticipatory pain relief dosing" before starting an activity. Taking pain medication immediately before the square dance isn't going to allow the comfort in movement you expect and desire, as it needs approximately 30 minutes to take effect.

As a general rule, all medications, no matter what category they fall in, should be used as prescribed and with caution. Even the most benign OTC medications can have disastrous side effects to the "at risk" patient. Sedation is a risk with most OTC medications. Therefore, caution should be used before starting tasks requiring vigilance and alertness until you are comfortable and familiar with your body's reaction to these medications. Do not drink alcohol with these medications and always update your physician as to changes in other prescription medications, in order to minimize the risk of side effects and medical interactions. Do not share your medications, in a call for empathy, with a friend or family member since there may be unknown risks from their own medical conditions. Recreational drug use, a growing concern in our adolescents and teenagers, has been found to be initially introduced through their parents' prescriptions. Therefore, be extremely diligent regarding your medication's storage and accessibility to others.

The narcotic lingo that you must understand is the difference between addiction, tolerance and dependence. The reality is that less than 1 percent of patients who were prescribed opioids for acute pain develop an addiction problem. "Addiction" can be viewed as a psychological dependence, with patients displaying cravings for narcotics, and an overwhelming involvement in obtaining and using them for reasons other than pain control. Quality of life is not benefited by the medication's use. These patients may miss work and run out of money due to the pathological use of the medications. This is in contrast to "tolerance", which is a need for escalating doses of the drug to maintain the same amount of pain relief. Usually, larger doses or more frequent use of the medication are needed over time, due to the liver enzymes "revving up" and metabolizing the narcotic. Due to this metabolic change, there may be less narcotic actually entering the bloodstream. The treatment for this may be "narcotic rotation," the use of another type of narcotic to which the body hasn't accommodated itself. Lastly, "dependence" is a response to chronic opioid use, characterized by the onset of acute withdrawal syndrome upon stopping usage. Classical withdrawal symptoms include flu-like symptoms, sweating, and diarrhea. People who are on chronic narcotic therapy (addicted, tolerant, or otherwise), may experience uncomfortable painful withdrawal. Therefore, for the above reason, abruptly stopping the use of chronic opioids should never occur, and a slow tapering off is most desirable and necessary.

CHAPTER 9

Diagnostic Tools

There are many different types of tests that your physician may request, in order to evaluate your pain syndrome. These consist of blood tests, electrical diagnostic studies, and radiological evaluations. For the most part, tests are rarely performed during the first few weeks of pain complaints, unless the discomfort is accompanied by other significant findings, such as searing and intractable symptoms, fevers, weight loss, night sweats, incontinence, or neurological losses.

Blood testing, most often performed by a concerned physician, may include a battery of basic labs that one undergoes for a routine physical. These include testing your blood concentration level, known as hemoglobin, as well as electrolytes, which reflect kidney function and hydration level. Sometimes, liver function enzymes are ordered for a more comprehensive evaluation. Marked abnormalities in any one of these lab findings may be a sign of a more significant problem that is manifesting as pain, and needs further medical evaluation. Cancer, with metastasis to the bones and liver, and with associated internal bleeding, is a common example of a disease process that can cause pain and abnormalities in laboratory blood work to be seen. In addition to these tests, inflammatory markers may also be ordered. These markers may indicate autoimmune disorders, infections or cancer. White blood cell count, sedimentation rate, and C - reactive protein are the most common inflammatory markers. Their elevation, by itself, has limited value, unless a source of their abnormally high level is found, such as osteomyelitis or infection in the bone. A rheumatologist may order more specific autoimmune markers, looking for other arthritic syndromes.

Electromyography and nerve conduction tests are ordered to learn more about the health of individual nerves. These tests help evaluate damaged or pinched nerves and approximate the severity and location of the damage along the course of the nerve. The results of this test are directly dependent upon the skill of the person administering and interpreting the study. A nerve conduction test is performed, quite simply, by putting a surface electrode lead, appearing similar to an EKG lead, over one part of the nerve and another lead over another part of the same nerve some distance away. The technician stimulates the nerve using an electric current through the first lead and measures the arrival of that electric current at the second lead. Based upon the current pattern seen from the second lead, we can interpret the health of the nerve. A healthier nerve will conduct faster, and with larger amplitude than a more compromised or pinched nerve. Repeat electro diagnostic testing may be performed annually to test for progression of neurologic dysfunction.

An EMG, or electromyography, is a measure of the health of muscles, compared to the prior test, which addresses purely nerve function. An EMG measures the electrical activity involved in muscle response to nerve stimulation. This is a very uncomfortable test, as it requires acupuncture-type needles to be placed into various muscle groups in order to record electrical signals. A healthy muscle has a pattern of electrical activity different from a diseased muscle. By using the nerve conduction studies and EMG studies together, a physician can differentiate a primary nerve disorder from a primary muscle disorder.

There is a large spectrum of radiologic testing one may order to evaluate different parts of the body. Of all the medical fields, radiology has seen the most significant strides in advancement over the past two decades, aided by breakthroughs in technology and in computers. I will touch on many of the basic radiologic tests that the patient may receive when undergoing an initial diagnostic work-up.

The range of studies varies from the simple x-ray to the more advanced 3-dimensional computer rendering of the human body using CAT scans or MRIs. As technology has advanced, these expensive techniques have been perfected and brought to the market, giving physicians an advanced ability to detect disease that would have otherwise gone undiagnosed. This, unfortunately, has led to higher medical costs, but the quality and need for these studies is a reality that no one denies.

X-rays are the simplest tool, and they show bone or other dense materials we purposefully place in the body. Barium is such a material placed in the gastrointestinal tract, with x-rays of the barium reflecting the passage of intestinal material. Narrowing of the barium in the intestinal lumen may reflect obstruction or tumor.

When it comes to the bones, the most common visualized x-ray abnormality is degenerative arthritic changes. This means, a narrowed disc space or bones showing signs of arthritic wear and tear as in knee arthritis. In reference to the spine, these changes are called "spondylosis", derived from the Greek word "spondylos", meaning "vertebra." Historically, many specialists noticing the degenerative spondylosis changes would point out that spot to the patient as their source of pain. However, more recent studies have shown questionable correlation between these x-ray abnormalities and the patient's pain complaint. Beginning at the approximate age of 18, there are degenerative x-ray changes in the spine, particularly the lumbar and the cervical areas. Over one-half of the population will show these changes by age fifty, making changes so common, that their help in diagnosis of pain syndromes becomes quite minimal. X-rays require exposure to radiation, having a cumulative effect over a lifetime. Therefore, especially in recent times, physicians and patients have been made more aware of avoiding excessive x-ray exposure for medical tests. Though x-rays hold invaluable medical information, one must realize that the largest disc herniation causing pain and neurological deficits will have a normal x-ray appearance, as this is a soft tissue abnormality and the disc is not seen in the bones visualized by x-ray.

Though x-rays are commonly used for bone evaluation, they also may be used to evaluate digestive problems. Plain, abdominal x-rays may show an obstruction or paralysis of the digestive tract leading to air-fluid levels. There also may be abnormal air patterns in the body cavity, indicating intestinal perforation or infection. Sometimes enlargements of the spleen, liver, and kidneys may be seen on x-rays. Barium studies use a cement-like material which is often swallowed to augment x-ray visualization of the intestinal tract, outlining the contours of the esophagus, small intestine, and the stomach. Abnormal patterns of barium in the intestine may signify tumors, ulcers, fistulas or obstructions. Sometimes a fluoroscope, or live continuous x-ray, is used to observe the barium flow. The live fluoroscopic x-ray will determine the intestinal contraction pattern and shed further light on any intestinal abnormalities that can cause pain. Barium is not pleasant tasting, and due to its viscosity, may cause some intestinal cramping. Barium taken orally or rectally by enema is excreted in the stool as a white chalky material. Barium can cause significant constipation if left in the intestines. Safe rapid elimination is recommended, usually through the use of oral hydration and laxatives.

CT scans (computed tomography) use x-ray in a computer-enhanced format, and is used to visualize any part of the human body. Unlike the x-ray, the CT scan uses a computer to generate two-dimensional, high-resolution images resembling anatomic slices of organs or of the brain. For a quality study, the patient must lie still for approximately 15 minutes. CT scans are better at reflecting bone than soft tissue pathology. A wide variety of bone, joint, and vertebral column abnormalities can be seen on CT scan. Intestinal abnormalities can be detected, especially when barium or some contrast medium is used. CT scans can also monitor the progression of disease by periodic scans and comparison with prior studies.

CT scans are sometimes used to detect heart disease by looking at plaque or calcium build-up in the coronary arteries. CT imaging also plays a role in viewing structural abnormalities of the heart, pericardium, major vessels, and lungs. Ultrafast-computer topography, a recent advancement (also referred to as cine-computed tomography) provides a three-dimensional, moving display of the heart, capable of detecting structural and motion abnormalities. A CT image requires the patient to lie upon a large gurney, which passes through an enlarged "doughnut hole" appearing device, which performs the elements of imaging. There is minimal sense of claustrophobia with these imaging techniques as compared to the MRI scan, which tends to involve a much narrower "doughnut hole" passage.

Magnetic Resonance Imaging (MRI) is undoubtedly the most sensitive form of imaging for screening for more serious pathology in the spine. Whereas a CT scan is a better technology to view bone pathology, MRI is a better imaging process to view soft tissue pathology, such as discs in the spine, or cartilage in the joints. It can reveal the state of the discs and the presence of protrusions or prolapses. It also can show detail in the spinal cord, nerve roots, facet joints, ligaments, and vascular structures. Due to the greater detail, MRI images take longer for a radiologist to study and report than a CT image.

Though the MRI is a great diagnostic tool, it may show too much detail in anatomy, leaving the physician with the dilemma of interpreting all this seemingly excessive information. Though invaluable when imaging disc pathology, there are often imaged "pathological wear and tear" disc changes in people who have never had any back pain. Therefore, when we see these same changes in patients with back pain, we question the significance of these findings. This is where technology and the patient can "clash", often requiring a good history and physical examination, from the astute physician, to put the entire picture together. Unfortunately, unsuspecting surgeons will operate on "pathology" with good intent and correct it surgically, but the patient will still have the initial pain problem. This may be a byproduct of too much advanced technology leading to a result that everyone wants to avoid-surgery; hence, the practice of medicine remains more of an "art" than a "science."

The main advantage of MRI scanning is that, there is no risk or harm to the patient resulting from x-ray exposure as used in the CT scan, in addition to better soft tissue imaging. The image is obtained by placing the patient in a narrow "doughnut hole" tube surrounded by large magnetic field coils, either in the upright or supine position. The body is composed mostly of water, and the magnet affects the hydrogen atoms contained in the water, orienting them along lines of a magnetic field. A magnetic current is then sent into the tissues, changing the orientation of all those hydrogen ions. When the current is stopped, the hydrogen orientation changes again, with a resulting discharge identified and processed as images collected in serial slices through the body. An accumulation of these sliced images will, via computer assistance, create a 3-dimensional picture. A CT scan is better at identifying small bone fractures or altered bone anatomy in comparison to more accurate soft tissue imaging using the MRI.

Myelography is a technique in which a CT or X-ray image of the spinal column is taken after injection of a radiopaque dye into the cerebral spinal fluid (CSF) within the spinal canal. Myelography can show abnormalities within the spinal column by showing blockage or abnormalities in the expected CSF pattern. In comparison to x-ray myelography studies, clearer images are obtained when a CT scan is used.

Most myelography has been replaced by the use of MRI images, capable of showing greater detail in the absence of spinal injection or radiation exposure. Myelography is usually now reserved for cases where previous spine surgery has been performed and the need to differentiate greater detail is needed. In these cases, a myelogram followed by a CT scan often gives more accurate image quality than an MRI in investigating the source of the pain. In cases where a patient has implanted electrical or metal devices such as cardiac pacemakers, MRI's cannot be used, due to the risk of disruption of the implanted device, and a myelogram with CT scan becomes a reasonable substitute.

Discography is used to diagnose the relevant disc as a source of pain. It is merely a diagnostic test and never therapeutic. Its accuracy as to determining if the disc is painful, and therefore the resultant decision for removal, is arguable. Some surgical colleagues would never remove and replace a patient's disc, or fuse their spines without a positive provocative disc injection study. Others don't view discography as having any predictive value in surgical outcome and make their surgical decisions based upon the anatomical MRI appearance.

Discography involves putting a needle into a disc at two or more levels. It is important to measure three different parameters during a discogram: 1) the patient's subjective report of pain (most important); 2) the radiographic appearance of contrast spread in the disc; and 3) the pressures within the disc as the contrast is injected. Through the needles and with the patient slightly sedated, we give a small amount of contrast and look at the radiologic appearance. If the contrast remains within the center of the disc, a result associated with elevated and sustained pressure measurements, this tends to be a healthy, non-painful disc. , when the contrast injected seems to spread throughout the disc and even leak out into the surrounding tissue or epidural space, this tends to be a sign of a degenerated disc with low pressures upon injection. Most importantly, the patient's self-report of pain on injection, seen with the degenerative disc, is the most valuable indicator of disc pathology. Surgical candidates are those that ideally have one "provocative" or painful disc that appears radiologically degenerated during discogram injection while the other discs are not painful. Poor surgical candidates are those that have provocative or painful discs at all levels tested, or no pain at any level tested.

A selective nerve root block is one that is performed to determine if a specific spinal nerve root is the source of pain. Sometimes there are many spinal areas of potential pathology, and the selective nerve root block helps identify the painful aberrant pathology from the non-painful. This procedure is done using fluoroscopic x-ray guidance with local anesthesia to allow patient comfort. The physician locates, via fluoroscopy, a specific spinal nerve root. The actual nerve root is not seen, as nerves are soft tissue, and therefore aren't seen using x-ray, but its location can be accurately inferred by knowledge of the surrounding bone anatomy. A needle is introduced through the skin into the area adjacent to the nerve root; medication is then injected into the area bathing the nerve root. These medications include an anesthetic and often, also a steroid. The relief of back and leg pain are the expected results which can last for weeks or months. If the pain relief is significant but short-lived and non-sustained, then a more permanent cure of surgical nerve root decompression can be reasonably entertained.

CHAPTER 10

Interventional Pain Management

Pain management is one of the newest, dynamic and exciting specialties in the medical world. It grew out of society's need for a physician to understand the complexities of pain, why it exists, how it affects the individual as a whole, and how to most effectively manage it. Prior to the pain specialist, an orthopedic physician would be knowledgeable in his sector, a neurologist in his, and an internist in his, et cetera; however, no one was able to put all the pieces together. A pain specialist who has interventional training is most highly touted, since his practice not only involves routine medical pain management, but interventional techniques used to augment comfort. Additionally, the pain management interventionalist is educated in disease processes, which in the past could only be referred to a neurologist, orthopedic surgeon, neurosurgeon, psychiatrist or internist to name a few. Clearly, pain management is an integrated multidisciplinary approach to pain control.

Everyone is aware of the unfortunate, runaway problem the medical community has with narcotic use in attempts to control pain. Interventional pain management is a specialty that may use medications and other disciplines to relieve pain, but primarily utilizes various injection techniques to avoid possible complicating factors associated with chronic, oral narcotic usage. Interventional pain procedures are performed in a setting allowing vital sign monitoring and fluoroscopic guidance - either in an office-based practice, ambulatory care center, or hospital outpatient center. The majority of procedures require 30 minutes or less to complete, and they are performed percutaneously (via needle insertion through the skin) under x-ray guidance by anesthesiologists skilled in these techniques. The need for sedation is variable, depending on the anxiety level and pain tolerance of the patient, as well as upon other coexistent medical problems. Though it is always nice to have sedation for interventional cases, it is not always practical or necessary.

The universal risks of bleeding, infection, nerve damage, headache, worsening pain, and seizures are commonly explained for these procedures, but highly unlikely to occur. The bleeding, infection, nerve damage, and worsening pain is from the insertion of a needle into the various parts of the anatomy, which can puncture blood vessels, introduce infection, traumatize nerves by direct contact or by the injected substance making the area briefly more swollen and painful. Extremely rare, seizures may occur as an adverse result of local anesthetic mistakenly injected in too high a dose or in an area that directly perfuses the brain. These seizures are generally fleeting.

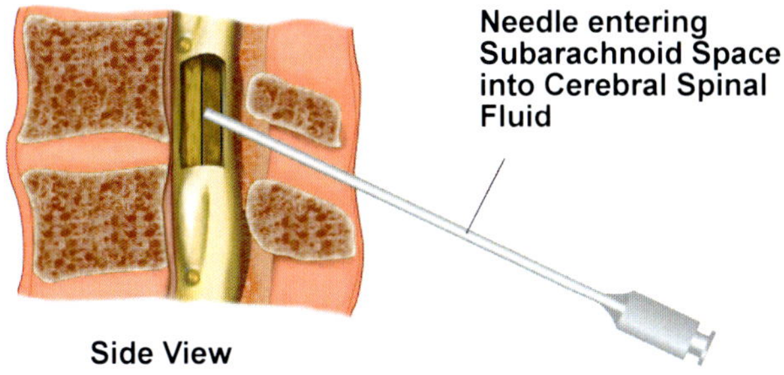

The most widely used intervention for acute disc herniation with nerve root impingement, is the epidural steroid injection. This herniation often leads to the development of radicular pain. "Radicular" comes from the Latin derivative of the word "root"; hence, it refers to an irritation of the nerve root. If the disc herniation is in the neck, then it often produces a cervical radiculopathy down the arm. If the disc herniation is in the low back or lumbar spine area, then it produces a lumbar radiculopathy down the legs. The epidural steroid injection is the most common injection given by the pain interventionalist, and is used for a variety of spine-related disorders including disc herniations, spinal stenosis, degenerative disc disease, spondylosis, spondylolisthesis and sciatica.

The epidural space is the space surrounding the spinal cord and nerve roots as they exit the spinal canal, traversing nearby the discs, before exiting out the bony foramen on their journey to the periphery. These injections can be given via various routes: caudal, translaminar or transforaminal. The injection is usually given under fluoroscopic x-ray guidance, to assure the needle is in the proper location. Contrast is often used, which acts like a dye that is visible on x-ray (fluoroscopy), to watch for flow of medication to the targeted pathological area of concern. Even though the needle may appear to be in a proper location, the contrast flow pattern is of paramount importance to evaluate for undetected injection into nearby blood vessels or spinal fluid. Epidurals associated with causing paralysis and permanent nerve damage are much more a myth than reality. Though there are rare complications, such as a hole, this procedure is performed routinely without a significant or frequent complication rate. The epidural steroid injection may function by two different mechanisms: decreasing swelling and irritation of discs and nerve roots, as well as washing away inflammatory substances that may exist in the epidural space.

The epidural steroid injection is usually given in an office- based practice or in an outpatient surgical area. No matter where the location, the physicians must have the proper licensing and credentials to practice this type of medicine in a safe and effective way. There is wide variation in the amount and type of local anesthetic used with the corticosteroid. This is all subject to individual practice bias.

Local anesthetic is often combined with the steroid in the injection syringe, to serve as direct feedback as to whether or not the target area has been reached. If properly placed, numbness and reduction of pain will occur within minutes after using the local anesthetic. The benefit from the steroid will not be immediate, unlike the local anesthetic, but instead may take several hours to many days to fully take effect. Therefore, many interventionalists wait one to two weeks between injections to fully assess their benefit. Complications from this injection rarely occur, but can include bleeding, infection, nerve damage, headache, local anesthetic toxicity, and allergic reactions.

Translaminar Epidural Steroid Injection

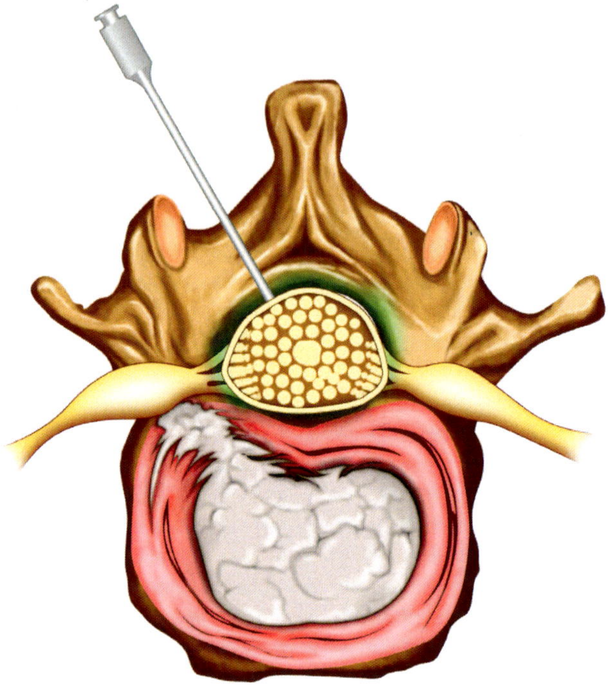

In the translaminar epidural steroid approach, also referred to as interlaminar, the needle is placed midline in the back and passed between the lamina of two adjacent vertebrae. The injection therefore targets mostly the posterior or back of the epidural space and then spreads to both the right and left sides. Use of contrast medium helps confirm appropriate spread before giving the steroid and local anesthetic.

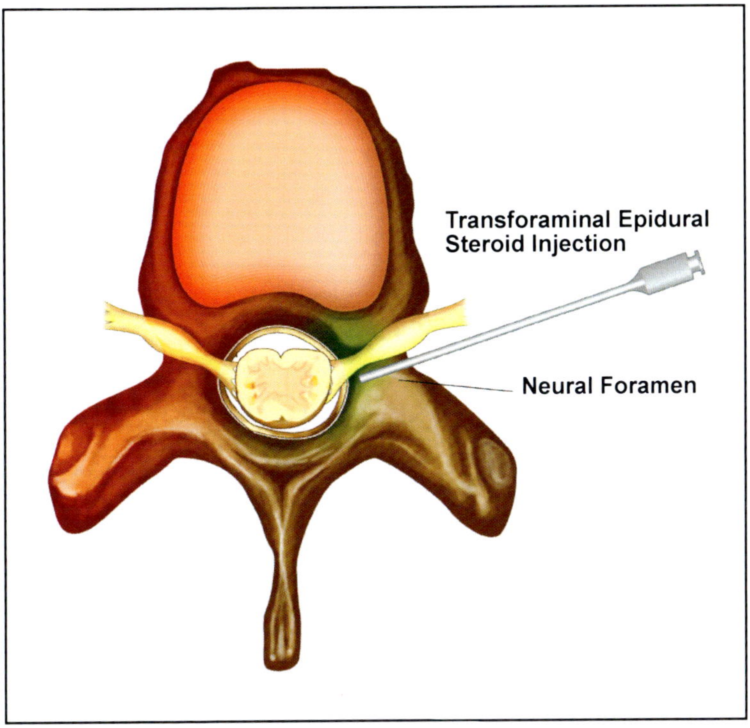

In the transforaminal epidural steroid approach, the needle is placed several inches to the side of midline and advanced into the neural foramen, adjacent to the exiting nerve root and in the most lateral aspect of the epidural space. Use of an injected contrast medium will confirm appropriate placement by its flow pattern. In the transforaminal epidural steroid approach, only one side or the other is targeted, therefore it is used most commonly for patients with unilateral or one-sided pain. It is also used in patients who have undergone previous spine surgery, thereby avoiding all the midline surgical anatomical changes such as residual scars, bone grafts, and fusion hardware. In the transforaminal approach, more so than with other epidural approaches, a brief paresthesia, or electrical "funny-bone" sensation, may radiate down the extremity due to the proximity of the needle to the exiting nerve root in the foramen. It is the most technically challenging epidural technique, but also often the most effective for unilateral pain. The transforaminal epidural steroid injection is used more hesitantly in the cervical and thoracic spine, due to concerns for damaging the blood flow to the spinal cord as the blood vessels enter through the foramen. This damage is more of a minimal concern in the lumbar area. In comparison, the translaminar approach can be used at any level of the vertebral column, though with greater caution above the lumbar spine, due to the existence of the spinal cord. Once injecting below the spinal cord level of termination, approximately L1, the risk of nerve damage is markedly reduced, since only individual nerve roots, and not the entire cord, is located below this level.

Caudal Epidural Steroid Injection

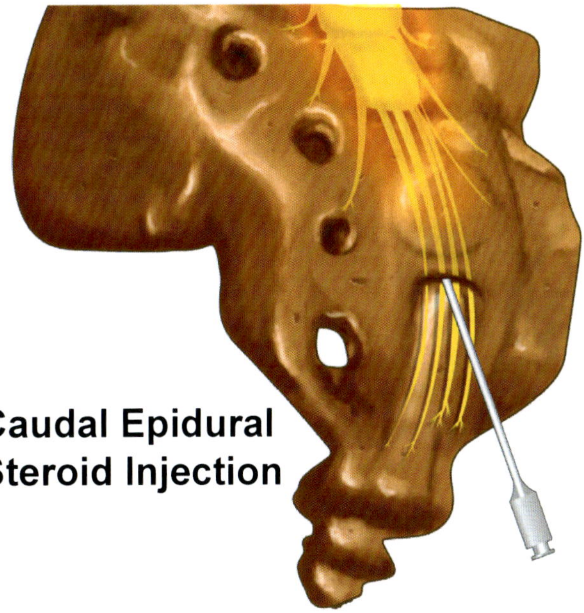

A caudal epidural steroid injection is placed in the midline of the tailbone area through a palpable foramen just above the gluteal, or buttock, crease. The needle is advanced, under x-ray guidance, to the upper sacral level. Injection at this level will reach only the sacral and lower lumber nerve root area. It may spread mostly to one side or to both sides in a "Christmas Tree" pattern seen on the fluoroscope, depending upon the orientation of the needle. Contrast, therefore, must be used to determine the flow pattern. The caudal approach also avoids any surgical scar or hardware issues similar to the transforaminal approach.

If needed, the breaking up of scar tissue caused by

previous spine surgery, referred to as "lysis of adhesions", can be performed through the caudal approach. This is accomplished using a semi-rigid catheter, seen under x-ray, which can be lodged into the scar. The injection of large amounts of fluid through this lodged catheter can break up the adhesions. The most recent technologies incorporate the same process of lysis of adhesions, but using fiberoptic scopes for better visualization of the anatomy, and lasers to destroy the adhesions.

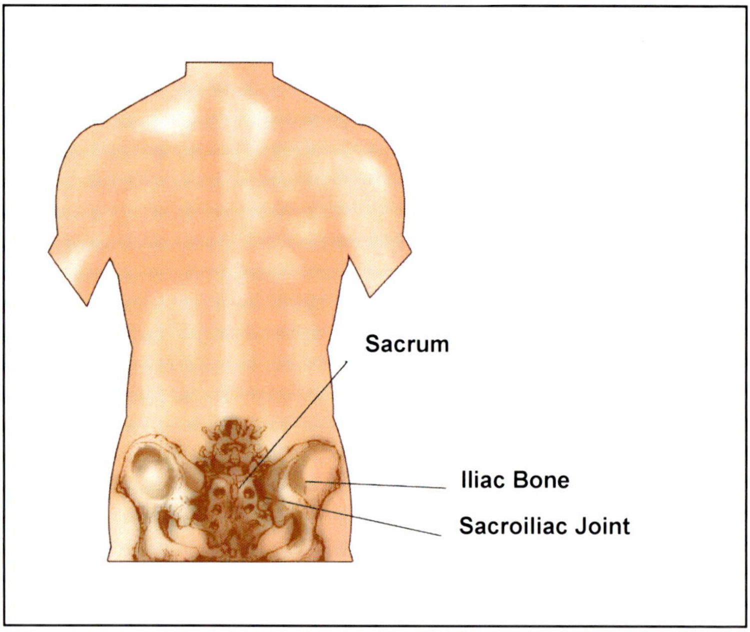

The sacroiliac (S.I.) joint is a propeller blade shaped joint lying on either side of the upper buttock area. S.I. injections are met with some controversy, as specialists are divided in opinion as to the frequency in which this joint is a pain generator. Certainly the joint is mobile in the younger patient, with the pregnant woman having the greatest joint laxity, allowing room for the baby's head to descend into the birth canal. The question exists, however, as to how often can the joint be a valid source of pain in the elderly. In the area of the S.I. joint, there are many other anatomical structures that can cause pain. These pain generators include disc degeneration, facet disease, and lumbosacral strain from surrounding muscles, ligaments and tendons. If pain is truly from the S.I joint, one must consider causes such as leg length discrepancies, hypermobility, trauma history, or recurrent sports and athletic injuries. Additionally, some rheumatologic diseases must be evaluated as they may cause S.I. joint arthritic pathology, which can also cause chronic sacroiliac joint pain.

The S.I. joint is easily identified using x-ray guidance, seen on either side of the sacrum. Injection is performed at the lower pole of the joint, as this is its most accessible area. Medication combinations, similar to the epidural medications, can be given into the joint. There have been some attempts to surgically fuse the joint with various degrees of success.

Facet joint blocks are performed because of localized pain, mostly in the back. Facet joints exist from the cervical down to the bottom of the lumbar spine and are pain generators to be evaluated in aching cervical, thoracic, or lumbar back pain. Facet joints do not cause radicular shooting leg or arm pain. The mainstay of their pain pattern is limited to areas around the spine and is often referred to as "mechanical" back pain. Since facet joints are in the back or most posterior aspect of the spine, arching backward, especially with twisting, and thereby compressing facet joints together can accentuate the pain and make it worse. This is called spinal extension, and it is one of the physical exam tests used to evaluate back pain. Tenderness on palpation of the facet joints, which lie on either side of the spine, can also aid in diagnosis. Unfortunately, research shows that there are no classical, reliable, physical exam findings from the facet joints. In other words, the exam could be negative, even though the facet joints were the cause of the pain. Likewise, the radiologic workup may show no abnormalities, even though the facet joints are causing this discomfort.

Facet joint blocks are done under x-ray guidance in a style similar to all other epidural or interventional techniques. The joints are easily visualized using x-ray. The actual facet joint may be injected or, the nerve to the joint may be blocked separately or in addition to the joint. This nerve is referred to as the medial branch, and comes off the nerve root as it exits the spine. It is easy to find, since it traverses certain bony spine landmarks easy to visualize under fluoroscopic guidance. Steroid and local anesthetics are injected into the joint, but most commonly, only local anesthetics are given at the nerve area. If the pain relief is excellent yet non-sustained, then a more permanent block using a radiofrequency probe targeting the medial branch can be performed. The risks of bleeding, infection, nerve damage, and headache, similar to the epidural, also exist with these procedures.

Lumbar Spine Discogram Symptomatic at L5-S1

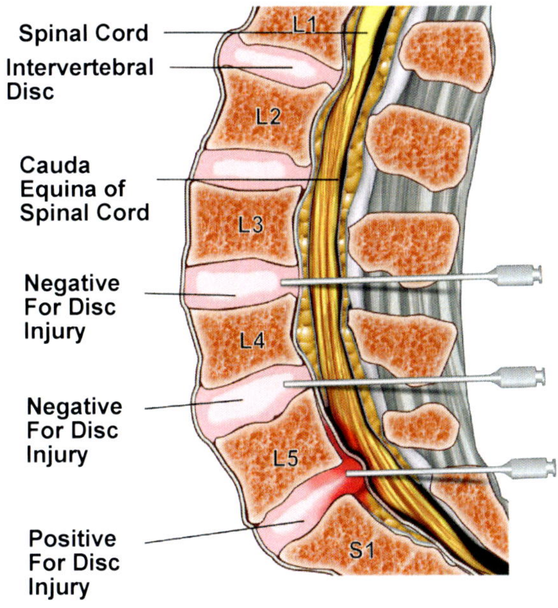

Another source of diffuse mechanical low back pain is from disc degeneration. This diagnosis cannot be confirmed solely by imaging such as MRI. The MRI may give a hint as to which discs appear narrow or markedly degenerated, but a direct disc injection to provoke and replicate the pain is most commonly pursued to confirm the disc as a pain generator.

This technique, performed under x-ray guidance, is reserved for patients with significant impairment and who have failed months of more conservative medical and interventional approaches. The discogram entails the percutaneous injection of a small amount of contrast medium into the center of the discs to see if the patient's typical pain is produced. The patient's subjective report of pain is the most important measurement criteria. Additionally, more objective criteria exist, such as the contrast pattern flow and the pressure required for injection. Usually the injection is performed at many different levels, with at least one being a "control"- a normal disc that should not be painful for the patient. If all discs injected are painful, then the patient is a less optimal surgical disc replacement or fusion candidate, as compared to the patient having only one painful disc. Not all surgeons or pain physicians place significant emphasis on the need for a discogram, as there are controversies over its predictive surgical value. However, to help find generators of non-specific low back pain which can have various origins, this diagnostic procedure may help clarify the disc as a source of non-specific low back pain before a large spine surgical procedure is agreed upon.

Trigger points are areas of tight, hyperactive bands of muscles located anywhere in the body, but usually in the back of the neck or low back. These "triggers" can exist primarily due to intrinsic muscle spasm or secondarily from spine related issues such as a disc herniation or nerve root impingement. For these secondary causes, the spasmodic muscle response helps prevent movement, hence decreasing the further experience of pain. Where there is no movement, there often is no pain. These are extremely rewarding and easy to treat as pain relief often occurs immediately. Acute trigger point pain development, occurring over several weeks, responds much more readily than chronic triggers existing for months to years. Prior to needle injection of these areas, more conservative approaches can be tried such as massage, ultrasound, and physical therapy.

A trigger point is very painful and may refer itself to other locations, mimicking a disc herniation with nerve root impingement. One example of "muscle pain" which can project to different areas is found in patients with angina from heart disease, as the heart is one big muscle. The pain from angina may be felt in the chest, or may only be described as jaw pain or pain with tingling and numbness down the arm. In the case of trigger points, the tense muscle will constrict its own blood flow, causing further pain due to muscle oxygen deprivation and the build-up of acidic waste metabolites. This pain, in turn, causes a spinal reflex system creating greater muscle tension and pain in a positive feedback loop process. Trigger point injections are most often performed in exam rooms using a small needle with local anesthetic, or sometimes by the needle alone. A distinctive, accentuated spasm and release may be noticed when the needle enters the correct area, hence the "trigger" of the muscle.

Sympathetic nerve blocks, most frequently targeting the stellate ganglion block in the neck, or lumbar sympathetic block in the low back, are used to block the sympathetic nervous system. The sympathetic nervous system, which is located outside and on either side of the spinal column, is the part of the nervous system that controls the body's "automatic" functions such as flow of blood, constriction and dilation of blood vessels, and temperature control. It is part of the larger category of the "autonomic nervous system", comprised of the sympathetic (fight or flight) and parasympathetic (rest and digest) responses, neither of which is under significant voluntary control. Some pain fibers, such as those involved in reflex sympathetic dystrophy (RSD), herpes zoster (shingles) and sympathetic pain syndromes, may travel through this sympathetic system or involve this system, requiring nerve blocks to minimize pain.

A lumbar sympathetic block is performed for pain syndromes that involve the lower torso or legs. As a result of blocking sympathetic fibers, the patient will have dilation of the blood vessels in the leg, which creates a feeling of comfortable warmth. In addition, there will often be pain reduction, decreased leg swelling, decreased color changes, and decreased sweating if it exists. The injection is performed under x-ray guidance with the patient lying on his abdomen (prone), similar to the position for epidural injections. It is performed on one side or the other, with the needle insertion site at least several inches to the side of the midline of the spine. The needle is advanced just in front of, and to the side of the spinal column, referred to as "anterolateral placement." Contrast medium is injected once again, to confirm appropriate placement. Local anesthetic is then given to block the surrounding nerves. The benefit from these injections may last hours to days, with a return of pain, but to a lesser baseline. Therefore, a series of injections may be performed until the pain is resolved, or "self-extinguishes."

A stellate ganglion block involves the same concepts, with similar indications and results as the lumbar sympathetic block. The stellate ganglion block involves the head and upper extremities instead of the lower torso and lower extremities, as with the lumbar sympathetic block. The stellate ganglion block is on either side of the cervical spine, and is performed with the patient lying on his back or supine. X-ray may or may not be used, depending upon physician preference. If no x-rays are used, there is no reason to inject contrast.

The celiac plexus is also part of the autonomic nervous system similar to the lumbar sympathetic and stellate ganglion nerve fibers. A celiac plexus block is commonly performed for abdominal pain, and is most often used to treat intractable pain of pancreatic cancer origin. It may also be used for pain due to pathology in the liver, gallbladder, stomach, kidneys, spleen, or certain areas of the intestines. Its location is in the upper mid-abdomen, just beneath the bottom of the lungs. The block is commonly performed with the patient lying on his abdomen while the needle is advanced towards the upper lumbar area, starting at a position several centimeters from the side of the spine. Alternatively, the procedure may be performed through the front of the abdomen, or via an anterior approach. Either way, the procedure requires x-ray guidance and contrast to confirm proper location. A large dose of local anesthetic is then injected to block the celiac fibers. In the case of pancreatic cancer, phenol or alcohol may be injected to permanently destroy the celiac fibers, thereby giving the patient more sustained relief.

Radiofrequency ablation is a percutaneous needle injection procedure which involves the creation of a nerve lesion produced by localized heat from radiofrequency waves. When the lesion is performed on a nerve sending pain signals, the pain transmission and perception by the brain is decreased. Various nerves throughout the body can be targeted for radiofrequency lesioning, although it is most commonly performed on autonomic fibers and medial branches of facet joints. The procedure uses x-ray guidance, with the added benefit of both sensory and motor stimulation through the needle to ascertain proper needle placement. There are two types of radiofrequency ablation: radiofrequency thermo-coagulation, which involves heating the tip of the needle to 80 degrees centigrade, and a milder, pulsed radiofrequency, which uses a lower temperature, "stunning" rather than destroying the nerves as seen in the higher temperatures. Pain relief from radiofrequency may not commence for several weeks after the procedure, but tends to last at least several months and can be repeated as needed.

Disc denervation is a radiofrequency ablation technique used for discogenic pain. Discogenic pain is back pain, commonly in the neck or low back, related to disc degeneration confirmed by a diagnostic discogram procedure. The discogram entails the placement of a needle into the painful disc and replicating the usual pain when a contrast agent is injected. The outside, or annulus of the disc, has a large amount of nerves surrounding it, and is therefore referred to as "highly innervated." Through heat generated by the procedure, the nerves involved in transmitting pain signals from the disc are destroyed; hence, the brain perceives no pain. The advantage of this procedure is that the duration and intensity of heat exposure is well controlled with minimal risk of damaging the nearby spinal cord or nerve roots. The duration of benefit is variable, anywhere from six months to two years, and may be repeated as necessary.

Occipital nerve blocks are injections used to treat pain conditions involving the back of the head, or occiput, with radiation towards the front, which are often associated with headaches. These pain conditions are formally referred to as "occipital neuralgia" and "cervicogenic headaches," the latter also being associated with cervical stenosis or arthritis in the cervical facet joints area, known as "cervical spondylosis." The occipital nerve block actually blocks two different neighboring nerves, the greater and lesser occipital nerves. These two nerves arise from branches of the 2nd and 3rd cervical nerve roots, traveling through the deep paraspinous muscles before becoming more superficial in the back of the skull going up the scalp.

The occipital nerve block is performed commonly without need for x-ray guidance. Since the nerve is located 2-3 inches from midline on either side of the scalp, it may be performed on only one painful side or on both sides (bilateral) if it is necessitated by the location of the pain. The physician often palpates the lowest part of the bony skull on either side of the midline, at times replicating the pain with pressure on the nerve with his fingers. Occasionally, an accompanying artery is felt pulsating nearby the location of the nerves. Since nerves are so active, requiring a lot of oxygen and nutrients, they are commonly found near blood vessels. A small needle is advanced towards the nerves and a local anesthetic is injected, sometimes combined with steroid, to anesthetize the nerve. Numbness to the top of the head and exquisite pain relief follows shortly thereafter. This is one of the procedures most gratifying to perform, since it gives patients tremendous relief: universally they go home smiling and thankful. The procedure may be repeated as necessary to give more permanent relief. If only non-sustained temporary relief occurs, then consideration is given to a radiofrequency procedure or an implantable electrical stimulation device; the latter is detailed in the next chapter.

Peripheral nerve blocks are injections into nerve bundles at a distance from the spinal cord. The most common example of this is an injection of the axillary nerve in the armpit in order to block all sensation and motor function distally in the arm and hand. These procedures are commonly done in operating rooms when only a single limb needs to be anesthetized for surgery. In the non-operating room setting, the procedure can be used to render a given part of the anatomy pain free or to allow a joint to be anesthetized and subsequently manipulated in a pain-free state. This manipulation, under anesthetic block, allows the breaking up of any joint adhesions or scars. Aside from axillary nerve blocks, other common peripheral blocks include interscalene, sciatic, and femoral nerve blocks. The technique is performed like the others, under sterile conditions and percutaneously, guided by ultrasound or x-ray. Sometimes the nerve block can be performed using a needle with an electrical tip, functioning to stimulate the muscles connected to that nerve, thereby confirming nerve contact. Various local anesthetics and their volumes may be used, which will determine if the block lasts for only one to two hours or as long as a full day if needed.

Kyphoplasty and vertebroplasty are both techniques incorporating the injection of cement into collapsed vertebral bodies, known as compression fractures, to alleviate pain, restore vertebral height, and prevent a domino effect of further compression fractures with the associated pathological, anatomical posture a patient would experience. The compression fractures are most commonly from osteoporosis, though in a minority of cases, a tumor may be responsible.

Vertebroplasty involves the percutaneous injection of cement into the vertebral body under X-ray control. Care must be taken that the cement doesn't leak out of the bone into other areas such as blood vessels or into the nearby spinal canal itself, which could compress the nerves contained within. In contrast, kyphoplasty involves a similar technique, but first a balloon is inflated in the vertebral body to form a cavity for the cement to follow. When the balloon first creates a cavity for the cement in this manner, there appears to be better control of the flow of the cement. These techniques are best performed when the fracture is acute, less than several weeks old. As time passes, the fracture becomes more permanently scarred and solid, therefore more resistant to reversal with cement under pressure. These procedures can remove pain immediately, though compression fracture pain does tend to diminish within several weeks to months, albeit with some postural kyphosis (leaning forward) due to compressed anatomy of the vertebrae.

As with all procedures, there is always a risk of complications, though rare, when these techniques are properly performed. Kyphoplasty and vertebroplasty are minimally invasive treatments for many who suffer from compression fracture pain. Leaking of cement outside the vertebral body is the greatest risk. This cement can spread into blood vessels, embolize to the lungs, or compress the nerves in the adjacent spinal canal. The use of x-ray is imperative to judge the spread of the cement as you expand the vertebral body.

For fracture prevention, strengthening bone to prevent further bone density loss is the objective. This can be accomplished by increasing exercise levels, weight lifting, calcium supplements, vitamin D and bisphosphonates such as Fosomax, which all function to reduce osteoporosis risks. Routine bone density measurements assist in judging the effectiveness of this treatment.

CHAPTER 11

Implantable Therapies

Implantable devices, including spinal cord stimulation (SCS) and intrathecal pumps (ITP) are the latest, cutting edge technology for people suffering with chronic pain. Both of these procedures involve simple outpatient trials first, testing for efficacy. If the trial is successful, then the patient is scheduled to return for permanent surgical placement of these devices. This necessitates the use of an operating room for strict sterile technique. The implants take no longer than a couple of hours and are performed through small incisions. Complications seen in both of these techniques, in the immediate postoperative period, are bleeding into the surgical site and infection of the hardware. Long term, there are risks of equipment failure, resulting in no pain relief. Rarely are there catastrophic consequences, unless there is an abrupt cessation of medication delivery through the pump. Psychiatric evaluation is required by most insurance carriers prior to a permanent implant procedure for pain control. Though patients often find this offensive, I assure them this is the request of their insurance carrier, not of the physician.

In regards to spinal cord stimulation, the procedure

is performed using minimal intravenous sedation and by the use of a simple epidural technique. Unlike the epidural steroid injection, spinal cord stimulation encompasses passing a paperclip width wire through the epidural needle while we ask the patient to report when they feel the pleasant electrical stimulation overriding their usual pain. Once they feel appropriate stimulation and relief, we leave the wire in that epidural location and remove the epidural needle. The patient is sent home with the wires coming out of the skin (which is bandaged) which are attached to a cell phone sized battery device. This device, often attached to a belt or kept in a pocket, allows the patient to turn the current on or off, and increase the amplitude of current as needed. Trials last for at least several days and up to a week. The patient must not get the wire insertion site or bandage wet, to minimize risk of infection.

If the trial is successful - gauged by patient comfort, then we perform the same procedure, but in a permanent fashion, including installation of a pacemaker- sized battery pack in an adjoining location, usually the gluteal or buttock area. The spinal cord stimulator wires are threaded, subcutaneously, from the epidural space into the battery pack. As an alternative to the percutaneous epidural wire (lead) implant, a larger "paddle lead" device, the width of the fifth finger, is placed via a small surgical incision into the epidural space. This implant decision is dependent upon the quality of pain relief during the trial. Once permanently implanted, there is nothing remaining externally. Women can even wear a bikini with no significant visual blemish. This is not a painful permanent procedure process and is accomplished under sedation in two hours or less.

The principle behind the spinal cord stimulator is the activation of nerves in the sensory input aspect of the spinal cord, also referred to as the dorsal or posterior aspect of the spinal cord. This results in a more soothing sensory electrical sensation, overriding the pain. This benefit occurs because pain nerve fibers are small, poorly conducting fibers and easily over-ridden by sensory input from large fibers such as those stimulated by the electrical impulses. An example of the slow pain fiber conduction is the pain experienced after stubbing one's toe. One can recall counting up to"3" after stubbing one's toe and cringing while waiting for the pain to occur. An analogy for explaining how the stimulator works is to view the actions we subconsciously perform after burning our finger on a hot stove: we blow on it, shake the hand, and pour cold water over it. These actions are all causing other sensory inputs into the brain, overriding the pain sensory input; they do not change the damage to the body tissue from the burn. This principle is referred to as the "gate control principle"; only a certain amount of input can get through the "gate" to the spinal cord and up into the brain. Thankfully, the pain fiber inputs are easily over-ridden, and thereby blocked by other non-painful sensory inputs.

Spinal cord stimulation is a widely accepted medical treatment, approved by the FDA and covered by insurance plans. Annually, 50,000 neurotransmitters are implanted worldwide with over 70% of these patients claiming pain relief, improvement in quality of life, and decreased reliance of pain medication. SCS is not a cure for pain, but it is an aid in making the pain more manageable and diminishing suffering. It is best used for patients suffering from radicular pain: pain shooting down their legs or arms. Though less effective, it can also be used for back pain. There are many diagnoses for which spinal cord stimulation can be tried, including failed back syndrome, spinal stenosis, degenerative disc disease, radiculopathy, complex regional pain syndrome (RSD), and peripheral neuropathy. The device is only implanted permanently if the trial is successful. With the permanent implant, the patient always maintains the ability to turn the device on or off and change the amperage, and hence the intensity of stimulation, as they wish.

Spinal cord stimulation is not for everyone and should only be tried after failure of a reasonable trial of pain medications, physical therapy, nerve blocks, and other therapies. In addition to the risks of bleeding and infection, which are common to most procedures, there are risks specific to the spinal cord stimulator, such as lead migration (causing a failure to stimulate the proper location over time), lead fracture, battery failure, or electrical connection failure. The stimulator should not be used while driving a car since the twist of your torso while looking beside or behind you may cause a distracting increase in stimulation, as body posture changes may affect the physical placement of the lead in the epidural space. Additionally, stimulators may set off metal detectors and security systems. Therefore, an identification card is given to implant recipients. As a whole, the benefits far outweigh the risks of spinal cord stimulation. These include complete patient control of the device, minimal surgery needed to implant, and excellent pain control.

The same spinal cord stimulator technology and equipment has recently gained popularity for the treatment of many causes of nerve-related pain and peripheral neuralgias, also called "peripheral nerve" stimulators. To accomplish this treatment, electrodes are placed via insertion through small subcutaneous needles, along the nerve paths of the pain. This strategically placed electrical lead will lie nearby the peripheral nerve and deliver low-level electrical impulses that interfere with the perception of pain, similar to its epidural mechanism of action. A four to seven-day trial of the peripheral stimulator is carried out with the electrical lead secured to the skin and then coming out to a battery pack that can be worn on the belt or kept in a pocket. This "trial lead" is then easily removed in the office, similar to an epidural trial lead removal. Permanent lead placement is performed in a similar fashion as the trial, but a battery pack, the size of a pacemaker battery, is also implanted under the skin at a nearby adjoining location. This implant is minimally detectable from external observation after the procedure is complete and healing has occurred. There are many centers now using peripheral nerve stimulation for craniofacial pain and other peripheral nerve syndromes because it's minimally invasive, can be trialed first, is reversible, and can be easily adjusted.

The final category for stimulator technology is referred to as "field stimulation". This is used for patients experiencing pain unable to be relieved by the placement of epidural or peripheral nerve stimulation. The usual location of this pain is in the back of the neck or lumbar area, both of them often refractory to the aforementioned stimulator strategies. The SCS lead placement is easily performed by placing two or more leads subcutaneously at the borders of the painful area and about 6 inches from each other. When the electrical current is applied, the separated leads "cross-talk", resulting in the patient experiencing a soothing sensation and not the prior pain. The permanent placement of these leads is quite simple as they are not located near critical structures, such as the spinal cord or peripheral nerves, as in previously discussed modalities.

Intrathecal Pumps (ITPs) are the other category of implantable devices also used in the treatment of many chronic pain states. They are used in treating a wide array of pathologies, including cancer pain, back pain, neuropathic pain and muscle spasticity. ITPs are automated pumps programmed to deliver medication into the cerebral spinal fluid (CSF) through a small catheter. This is a recent and exciting innovative technique, both safe and effective, especially since revolutionary new medications are being developed for use in these pumps.

The pump's role is to deliver pain medication directly to the CSF- the fluid surrounding and bathing the pain receptors in the spinal cord. By this direct delivery approach, smaller doses of medication, as compared to the oral route, are required to gain the same or even better pain relief. When oral pain medications are taken, they require processing in the stomach, bloodstream uptake, and then significant metabolism in the liver. After this all occurs, there has to be enough remaining to reach the target location of the pain receptors. ITP implants succeed by bypassing all this and putting medications, undiluted, exactly where needed: at the nerves transmitting pain signals from the spinal cord. It is a technique considered when oral pain meds and other methods of pain control have been exhausted, or proven ineffective due to excessive side effects.

Before the decision is made to implant an ITP, an intrathecal medication trial is performed by a simple spinal injection of the same medication, and then the patient is observed both for pain relief and side effects. Permanent ITP placement is achieved in an operating room using sedation with local anesthesia or general anesthesia. The permanent procedure involves a spinal needle being placed into the spinal canal as a conduit for a spinal catheter, then entering into the spinal canal using x-ray guidance. Once the catheter is in the proper location and secured, the spinal needle is removed and the pump is connected. It is placed subcutaneously in the lower abdomen. The catheter and pump are tunneled under the skin and the wounds are closed surgically. The entire procedure takes less than two hours on an outpatient or inpatient basis. The pump, via the connecting catheter, delivers pain medications at a rate of a fraction of a drop continuously and daily into the cerebral spinal fluid (CSF) around the spinal cord. The medication pump reservoir is easily and percutaneously, refilled every four to six weeks.

ITPs can be used to treat a variety of painful conditions including nociceptive pain (tissue injury), neuropathic pain (nerve injury), and spasticity. Nociceptive pain most commonly responds to the use of morphine at 1/300th of the dose required orally, thereby eliminating many of the oral narcotic side effects. Neuropathic pain may respond better to intrathecal local anesthetics or other medications that are not narcotic based. Common examples of neuropathic pain include complex regional pain syndrome or reflex sympathetic dystrophy, phantom pain, post herpetic neuralgia (shingles), failed back surgery syndrome, cancer pain, and peripheral neuropathy. Spasmodic pain can also be successfully treated with ITPs by using anti-spastic muscle-relaxing medications like Baclofen.

Spasticity - an abnormal increase in muscle tightening or tone, is the result of brain or spinal cord injury from various causes including stroke, spinal cord trauma, cerebral palsy, and multiple sclerosis. Baclofen, available orally, should be tried intrathecally only when significant oral doses fail due to the common side effect of sedation.

Intrathecal pump implants are effective and safe devices to use, but have some initial side effects that should be watched closely, depending upon the medication used in the pump. These side effects include sedation, weakness, itching, stomach upset, and respiratory depression. More serious complications to watch for are bleeding into the surgical wound, infection, meningitis, granulomatous mass formation around tip of the catheter in the CSF, and catheter or pump malfunction.

As a whole, ITPs are widely successful as are their spinal cord stimulator implantable counterparts. They allow for greater motor function and cognitive abilities when used for pain, and markedly reduce muscle tightness when used for spasticity. Both of these technologies, SCS and ITPs, are to be used only after a long and comprehensive look at the patient's medical history to insure that all of the more conservative modalities have been maximized. They are very effective in the correct patient candidate and are associated with an acceptably low side effect profile.

CHAPTER 12
Surgery

Undergoing spinal surgery is a big decision. It should be performed only after careful and detailed discussion with your surgeon regarding the risks and benefits. We all have friends who have undergone spine surgery and done remarkably well and others who received only short-term benefit, or unfortunately, those who are now worse. Surgery may be performed for various reasons. One reason is pain relief. More commonly it is performed for weakness or numbness in the arms or legs which may be associated with pain. Often times, patients may have a normal radiologic workup, including x-rays and MRIs, but still complain of pain; these patients are not operative candidates. Alternatively, there could be severe stenosis or a large disc herniation in the complete absence of pain or deficits. Patients with these findings are also not operative candidates. This variation in clinical scenarios frequently makes the pain diagnosis elusive and the surgical decision to operate more complicated. This common enigma emphasizes the reality of medicine being more of an “art” than purely a “science”. As a general rule, surgeons are more likely to operate for spinal conditions causing radicular leg or arm pain, especially when with associated neurological deficits. This is usually the result of stenosis or disc herniation seen on MRI. The results from operating on this radicular pain are overwhelmingly favorable in comparison to a less optimal outcome in operations for back or neck pain, independent of severity.

Patient education is essential before any surgical venture, to explain the intricate anatomy and reasons for pain. An educated and well-informed patient is capable of making a wiser decision and tends to have a more reasonable acceptance of the outcome, whether good or bad. Surgery leaves behind some scar and changes the spinal anatomy, even in the best of hands. As a result, the spinal anatomy is never "normal" again. Though surgery can be curative of pain in some conditions, in other conditions there may be less remarkable results. These conditions include slowly progressive chronic states, such as multi-level spinal stenosis. Surgery may partially reverse the problem or simply arrest further deterioration in neurological function, but will not give a pain-free cure.

Though spine surgery is often the last choice after more conservative measures have been tried, certain emergencies that need urgent surgical intervention include nerve or spinal cord compression from tumor, bleeding, or infection. Heightened attention should be given to patients "at risk" for these spine surgery emergencies: those with a history of cancer, those immunocompromised, or patients on anti-coagulants such as Plavix (clopidogrel bisulphate) or

Coumadin (warfarin). Patient complaints that should trigger urgent evaluation and surgical treatment include sudden onset weakness in the arms and legs, numbness in the anal or genital area, or rapidly progressive and intractable pain in the back or neck.

Anatomy was reviewed in a prior chapter, and we will review it again here in terms of the surgical approaches needed. The spine is divided into four different anatomical regions, each with unique properties due to location. We start from the top with the cervical spine (neck), followed by the thoracic spine, lumbar spine (low back), and tailbone area, also called the sacral and coccygeal region, located at the lowest region.

4 Divisions of the Spine

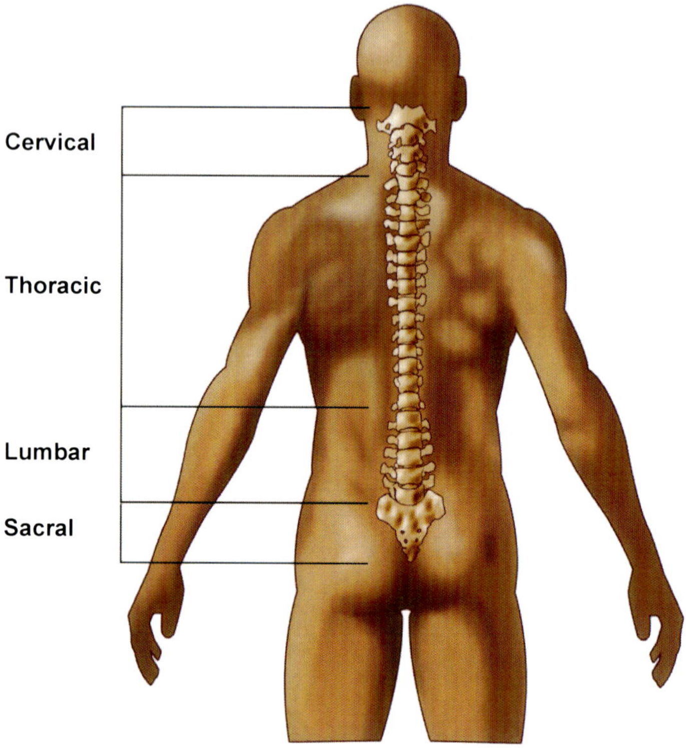

The neck contains seven vertebral bodies which are numbered C1 to C7. Each vertebral body has a disc above and below it, except for the highest levels. The discs are numbered depending upon the levels between which they fall. For example, a C5-6 disc is in-between the C5 and C6 vertebral bodies. Most of the cervical disc problems occur at the lower cervical levels because that is the same area responsible for all the motion. As a rule of thumb, where there is no motion, there is usually very little degeneration.

The thoracic spine has twelve vertebrae, each separated by a disc similar to the cervical and lumbar spine. Unique to the thoracic spine is that each vertebra is attached to the ribs. Due to the inherent stability that the rib cage provides for the thoracic vertebrae, there is very little motion in this area. This is an excellent design, as you would not want to have twisting and bending in your thoracic spine, putting you at risk for compressing the heart and lungs in that vulnerable area. Due to this relative lack of motion and hence, "wear and tear" of the thoracic spine, the problems of disc degeneration or spinal stenosis rarely develop. This is in contrast to the cervical spine above, and lumbar spine below, both being exposed to significant degenerative complications.

The lower back, or lumbar spine, consists of five vertebral bodies, each separated by discs. The disc between the thoracic and lumbar spine is referred to as the T12-L1 disc. The lowest disc separates this lumbar area from the sacral region and is referred to as the L5-S1 disc. There is significant degeneration which can occur throughout the entire lumbar spine, especially the lower lumbar area. This exists due to the weight bearing of the higher levels, all bearing down upon it, as well as significant motion which occurs with bending, lifting, sitting, etc. The overwhelming majority of spine surgery involves this area.

Sacral Spine - Side View

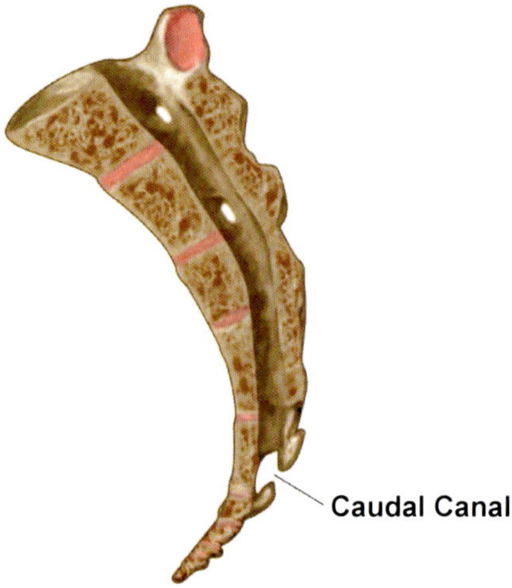

Sacral Spine - Posterior View

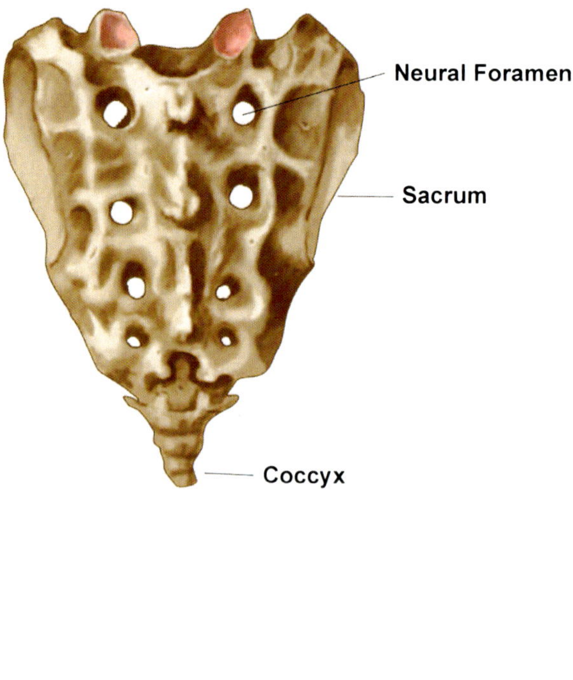

The tailbone consists of bones from the sacral and coccyx area. This is a unique area in the spine as there are no discs between these small bones. The bones are fused in a fashion with "seams" between each, but no true discs. The spinal nerve roots exit through boney foramen here without risk of impingement by disc herniation. Due to the relative lack of motion and no discs, there is almost no degeneration that can lead to nerve root impingement. Sometimes, a traumatic fall can cause a contusion or small fracture in an area resulting in lingering pain due to bruising. This does not need surgery and is best handled by patience, time, medical management and occasional localized injection.

The discs are the cushion-like shock absorbers between each vertebral body. The discs and vertebral bodies get larger in order to handle the progressive increased weight load as you go from the uppermost cervical regions down to the lumbar area. The disc structure can be compared to that of a "baked" jelly donut. The outside casing is called an annulus and the jelly inside is called the nucleous pulposis.

The facet joints are outcroppings or articulating processes from each vertebral level, almost like "antlers" which go upward and downward. There are two joints per level, one set on the right and the other on the left. They are labeled based upon the level with which they are associated, for example, the right L1-2 facet joint. These joints have many functions, which include keeping the spine in "check" to prevent excessive twisting, as well as functioning in a weight-bearing capacity.

The spinal canal, which exists at each vertebral level from the upper cervical spine to the tailbone, functions as a well protected boney conduit, housing the spinal cord and nerve roots. The nerves themselves lie within a fluid sac, called cerebral spinal fluid (CSF), contained in the spinal canal. The CSF keeps the nerves buoyant, protected, and also offers some nutritional value. One pair of nerves, one right and one left, exit the spinal canal at each vertebral level. As they exit, they leave the roomy comfort of the vacuous spinal canal and exit through small holes, or foramen, in the spinal canal on their way to the periphery. In their departure from the relative security of the spinal canal, they become peripheral nerves and are more vulnerable to disc or arthritic compression.

The spinal cord, a thick rope-like bundle of nerves, begins at the brainstem and descends, ending in the upper lumbar spine L1 level, sending off individual nerve roots at each level as it descends. Therefore, injury to the spinal canal above the first lumbar vertebrae, due to trauma or surgery, can injure a vast array of nerve fibers in the spinal cord bundle. Lower than L1, the cord no longer exists in the canal. The nerves are found individually in an array looking like a horse's tail, hence the description of the "cauda equina", and are associated with a lower risk of nerve injury with trauma or surgery. This anatomical change at L1 can be easily seen on an MRI scan.

Surgical discectomy to remove disc herniations is the most common spine surgery, and usually occurs at the lumbar level of the spine. It is performed when all other reasonable and conservative measures have been exhausted, including physical therapy, medical management, and other various interventional techniques. Time is a key factor with disc herniations. Some recent studies looking at patients with lumbar disc herniations show that those treated non-surgically or surgically have the same results at a two year follow-up. Needless to say, there are some controversies over the specific parameters of these studies, exclusion and inclusion criteria, etcetera. The existence of profound neurological deficits is an affirmation of an urgent need for surgery when compared with pain in the absence of deficits. For the rare, large disc herniations resulting in an unstable gait or incontinence, rapid surgical intervention is undoubtedly required. When it comes to spine surgery, most patients will not need to make a hasty decision, and will have the option of giving it more time or choosing to undergo surgery after understanding the inherent risks.

The two main categories of spine surgery are a decompression (including discectomy and laminectomy) and a fusion. Sometimes you can have both performed simultaneously due to anatomical and structural needs. Decompression is designed to remove disc or bone from impinging on the spinal cord or nerve roots. Discectomy is a decompression by removal of the disc material whereas a laminectomy is a decompression by removing part of the boney spinal canal which acts as a "cover" or "lamination" covering the cord and nerve roots. The fusion is performed because there is movement or instability of the spine, with resultant pinching of the nerves. Fusion can also be performed because of severe disc degeneration and no cushioning between each vertebral level. This lack of cushioning causes vertebral bone-upon-bone contact, which is very painful. Fusing this level will halt any bone-on-bone movement and subsequent pain. More recently, fusions are losing popularity to the cutting-edge, motion-sparing disc replacement surgery. By replacing the pathologic disc with a motion-preserving artificial one, there is prevention of degeneration of neighboring spinal segments (adjacent level disease), often seen after fusion.

The surgical gold standard for the treatment of disc problems remains the simple discectomy or microdiscectomy. This surgery involves general or spinal anesthesia and a small incision over the affected area. The surgeon cuts through the tissue to the disc which is identified visually and by x-ray confirmation. Depending upon patient and surgical influences, this surgery is often performed in less than 2 hours. The microdiscectomy wound is small, less than a couple of inches, and the patient experiences very little post-operative pain. Patients usually return home within 24 hours. This is a very satisfying surgery as it is quick and has minimal recovery period; most patients do quite well in long-term follow up.

There are other approaches to a simple disc herniation. This grouping is referred to as "percutaneous discectomy". This involves one of many different technologies. You approach the disc by a small skin incision followed by the advancement of a small "trocar", or straw sized device, to the level of the disc, using x-ray guidance. Through the trocar, you may advance a needle into the disc and inject chemical substances that shrink the disc. Alternatively, you may use a laser or radio frequency wave to ablate and shrink the disc, or possibly mechanically pull some disc material out. These are some of the newer technologies with indications and results still not formally agreed upon.

Lumbar Laminectomy

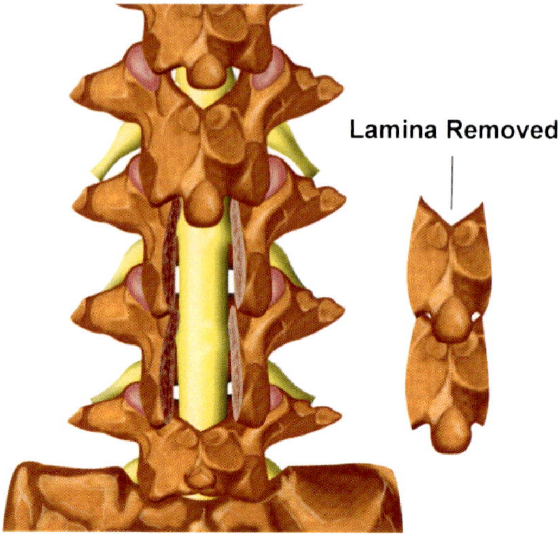

Surgical laminectomy to treat spinal stenosis involves removing some of the bone covering the spine. It is a more involved decompression procedure than the simple discectomy. Spinal stenosis is the disease of the more geriatric population and results from degenerative changes causing disc space narrowing, ligament overgrowth, and the development of arthritic bone spurs which narrow the spinal canal and exiting foramen. The result of this is "neurogenic claudication" or pain in the legs when walking, often relieved with rest or leaning forward, such as over a shopping cart. The pain when walking is often associated with loss of balance or loss of leg control. I see many of these patients in the local malls walking from one bench to the next, sitting at each before moving on.

Spinal stenosis with MRI evidence of one or two level impingement may be amenable to surgical laminectomy decompression. The lamina, or covering of the spinal canal, is similar in concept to the lamination of a tabletop. The more levels involved, the lower the success rate of the surgery. Epidural injections, medical management, canes or other ambulatory assistance devices should be attempted before deciding on surgery on these often frail and older patients. Surgery entails removal of part of the laminar bone, which is the covering of the spinal canal, to decompress this area. This allows CSF fluid and blood back to the previously severely compressed nerves. Since the lamina functions to support the spine, the surgeon cannot remove too much, as this would adversely alter spinal anatomy, possibly diminishing its inherent structural stability, causing spinal instability. This may call for the need of yet another surgery, spinal fusion.

A process detected on x-ray of one vertebral body sliding back or forth upon another is referred to as "spondylolisthesis" and occurs in about 5% of back pain patients. This is often degenerative in nature, occurring in people over the age of 50. Often it is a minor "slip" and causes minimal irritation to nerve roots or impingement on the canal. With age, these slips most commonly do not progress and rarely necessitate surgical fusion. For more advanced slips, as diagnosed on x-rays using flexion (bending forward) and extension (bending backward) views, there may be a significant component of instability needing surgical fusion with bone or hardware.

Spine surgery is performed by going through the front (anterior) aspect of the body, or the back (posterior). For most cervical spine surgeries, the anterior approach is used; however, large cervical fusions may necessitate a posterior approach. For thoracic spine surgeries, a posterior or lateral approach is often used. This is complicated, as it involves splitting ribs and working inside the chest cavity. The anesthesia for this is quite intricate. The surgical side lung is collapsed to allow exposure to the spine, so single lung ventilation is needed. Thankfully, since the thoracic spine is so inherently stable, surgery in this area is not common. Lumbar surgery may be performed posteriorly, which is most common, especially for disc removal, or anteriorly and posteriorly for more aggressive fusions.

One of the most serious complications of spinal surgery is infection, though each surgical approach has other unique complicating risks. Infection might have devastating consequences and often requires long-term intravenous or oral antibiotics. Infections may occur immediately or may not be detectable for several weeks or months after the surgery. The patient usually complains of worsening pain or even neurological problems. Fevers and redness in the surgical area are not reliable indicators of infection.

Laboratory work looking at inflammatory markers as well as radiologic workup must be pursued. Surgically opening the operative site to "wash out" the infected area and to obtain cultures may often be needed. Sometimes, leaving the surgical wound partially open with drains, frequent dressing changes, and irrigation are the best ways to resolve the infection, though admittedly unsightly. Hardware such as surgical plates and screws, commonly referred to as "foreign bodies", may make it especially difficult to clear the infection, as they have no natural blood supply and tend to harbor infections readily. Sometimes they may need to be removed in order to formally clear the infection.

Nerve damage may also be a complication of surgery. I see it most commonly as a result of prolonged nerve entrapment due to spinal stenosis or disc herniation, resulting in nerve damage that the surgery is intended to cure. Sometimes surgery incompletely reverses this pre-existent damage, resulting in some persistent residual pain. Nerve damage can occur as a direct consequence of surgical cutting, or due to the scarring and subsequent entrapment of nerve roots, which is part of the normal healing process. Headache may also sometimes occur if the CSF- containing fluid sac is inadvertently cut into.

Bleeding is yet another known complication, not only of spine surgery, but of all types of surgeries. The bleeding may cause a large, painful clot accumulation and may leak out of the surgical dressing. It will cause pain due to its mass and expansion into surrounding tissues. Unique to the spine though, is that bleeding into the wound may cause compression on the nerve roots or spinal cord, resulting in permanent nerve damage if not quickly noticed and surgically decompressed. Patients on blood thinners or who have kidney disease, liver disease, or coagulation defects are more prone to this.

Even with the best surgeon and patient, complications do arise. This is an unfortunate, but known and acceptable risk of the surgery. Treating complications by proper identification of the cause and having an agreed-upon plan is imperative. Sometimes the surgery cures one problem, but may cause another down the road. This is referred to as "adjacent level disease." An example of this would be the fusion of one painful level, which results in the adjacent spinal level now needing to be more mobile to compensate for the neighboring fused level. This previously normal level now becomes pathologic and degenerated due to the increased motion. For this reason, the more recent technology is motion-sparing surgery, such as artificial disc replacement instead of fusion. By allowing motion to continue uninterrupted, adjacent level disease is less likely to occur, especially in younger surgical patients. Allowing motion to continue uninterrupted prevents a cascade of spine surgeries to be required in the future.

Sometimes patients develop severe back pain in the absence of leg involvement. This can be from a degenerated disc which can then send pain signals. An MRI will often show evidence of disc pathology. A discogram, which is a percutaneous injection into the disc, can help further diagnose this. During the discogram, contrast is given at several disc space levels under pressure. If the patient has replication of the usual pain with injection, especially if it's associated with the contrast leaking out of the disc and lack of pressurization, then this helps confirm the pathological pain state of the disc. If the disc space height is maintained, an IDET (Intra Discal Electrothermal Coagulation) can be attempted, via percutaneous needle approach, to help make the nerves to that disc less sensitive. This is accomplished by placing a wire into the disc via the percutaneous needle. This wire coils around inside the disc and is heated by an electrical current. This destroys some of those small pain nerve fibers infiltrating the disc, hence making the patient more comfortable. It does not affect the anatomy of the disc and does not change the disc's appearance. However, if the disc space is markedly narrowed or collapsed, the patient becomes more of a candidate for a surgical fusion or replacement. Risks of the IDET procedure are failure to obtain pain relief (30%), infection (1%), nerve damage, and eventual need for surgery.

Posterior Lumbar Fusion

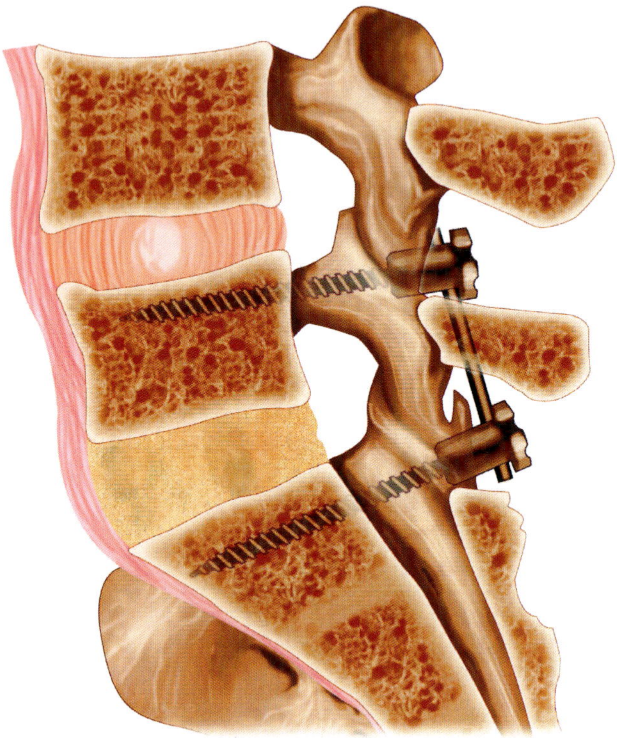

A fusion is the most substantial and serious form of the commonly performed spine surgeries. It has many indications and is most commonly performed for spinal instability or intractable pain from a disc degenerative source, termed discogenic pain. By definition, with a fusion you are fusing two or more vertebral bodies together, hence preventing motion at that level. Where there is no motion or movement there should be no pain, just like when you immobilize and cast a fractured bone in the arm. The role of the disc, at that level, will become nullified. In the case of discogenic pain involving one disc, the disc should be removed and replaced at that level or fused. If two or more discs are involved, the procedure is more aggressive, and usually involves a multi-level fusion with bone and hardware, typically plates and screws. Similarly, in the case of spondylolisthesis, or a slippage of the vertebral bodies to the point of causing nerve impingement, a fusion should be performed at the affected level. The fusions are most commonly done from the back, but may also require an anterior abdominal approach.

There are many ways to perform a fusion. They may be performed from the back, front or even through trocar-type, minimally invasive techniques. There may be plates and screws, which are affixed to the spine in order to prevent motion. There also may be devices placed in the disc area which achieve a fusion. Sometimes bone alone, in the absence of foreign body hardware, is used to accomplish this fusion. As a whole, fusions are far less successful for back pain than for pain associated with problems of nerve root impingement with resulting in pain radiating to the extremities.

The common complications are similar to previously discussed spine surgeries. These include nerve damage, bleeding, infection, and failure to achieve pain relief. Fusion failures are common amongst smokers due to the nicotine causing small blood vessels to constrict, which prevents healing. Many surgeons will refuse to operate on smokers due to this well-known complication. Sometimes, especially on thin people, the hardware may be close to the skin and cause pain, necessitating its removal. This usually happens many months or years after the surgery, so that hardware removal does not cause problems, since the secondary bone fusion has already occurred. Having MRIs with fusion hardware in place is safe. If the MRI is done at the level of the hardware, there may be a lot of "scatter" and low quality of visualization limited only to that immediate area. By the way, the fusion hardware will not set off store or airport security systems.

Chapter 13

The Fundamentals of Health Insurance

Choosing health-insurance has always been one of the most crucial purchases. As it is said, health is wealth; nothing is more important than protecting your health and having the most appropriate treatment under all circumstances. Therefore, the right time to buy health insurance is before you experience an injury, severe sickness, or mishap of any sort. When health insurance is purchased, it is only responsible for the coverage of medical treatment regarding the health problems faced after the policy is issued, unless special provisions are made for pre-existing conditions. For every individual, having essential knowledge relevant to health insurance is extremely useful.

As of this printing, there is no requirement under any state or federal law for your private employer to provide health insurance to his employees. However, a number of employers offer health insurance services in order to attract the most qualified and capable employees. If group health policies are provided, they are passed through state-authorization, concerning the type or nature of benefits that are required, except for situations in which the employer has a self-insurance policy. This means that the employer assumes the costs of the medical expenses.

Undoubtedly, health insurance state and federal mandates play a key role in broadening the coverage. However, oftentimes it increases the cost as well. For instance, according to the estimation of the Council for Affordable Health Insurance (CAHI), addition of coverage for birth control further increases the cost of a group health policy by 1 to 3 percent. State-mandated benefits are not applicable to individual (private-market) plans that are self-purchased.

When job changes or unemployment are present, the employee looks for a means to bridge the insurance gap until health insurance coverage resumes by the future employer. The federal COBRA law (Consolidated Omnibus Reconciliation Act) could possibly offer an employee limited time extension of benefits. COBRA enables workers to keep their group health coverage when job loss occurs, on the condition that full payment, including the administrative fee, is paid by the worker. It is applicable to those firms that have 20 or more employees and extends for around 18 months. It can be quite expensive to purchase continued coverage through COBRA.

HIPAA (Health Insurance Portability and Accountability Act) is another federal law that provides security to workers who change their group health policies. This law enforces regulation on the level to which certain group health plans can eliminate coverage for conditions that already exist. For example, if an individual has a history of "commendable" health insurance for 12 straight months, without any lapse in coverage for 63 days or more, a new group health plan must cover your previous conditions. Coverage of the medical problems is guaranteed once the enrollment in the plan is complete. Short-term health insurance and catastrophic health insurance are some of the alternative methods applied to purchasing health insurance when an individual is in between group health policies.

If (due to any reason) you are unable to purchase group health insurance through work, you may opt for a private-market health policy (also called the "individual health plan"). When talking about group plans, the expenses and hazards linked to health care are spread among many people, thereby averaging the liability. On the contrary, individual health insurance is "medically underwritten", taking into consideration the patient's health record, profession, age and sex. Conditions that already exist, including cardiovascular disease, diabetes and even pregnancy can bar you from being accepted, or cause an increase in the premium. Certain states want individual health insurers to provide each individual with a policy, irrespective of medical conditions - a mandate called the "guaranteed issue."

After you have opted for an individual health policy, your premiums may be changed. Usually, health insurance companies look for authorization to increase premiums. Furthermore, certain states permit health insurers to "file and use" rate boosts, meaning that the insurers have to submit a request for increase, which is usually approved. However, the state insurance commission may deem the increase excessive and negate the increase. Colleges play a significant role in obtaining sensible health insurance for their college students. There are a number of federally-sponsored programs to assist the student if the premiums are unaffordable for the individual, regardless of the student's age.

There are a number of government-sponsored programs available to members of the population meeting certain criteria. Medicare is a federal health insurance plan for individuals who are aged 65 and older, and for younger patients having disabilities, or those suffering from end-stage kidney diseases. Medicaid is a program designed for low-income families based upon IRS poverty levels. Each state handles its own citizens. State Children's Health Insurance Program (SCHIP) is a health care plan designed for children whose parents earn enough to be considered eligible for Medicaid, but their wages are not sufficient to satisfy the affordability requirements for individual health insurance. Certain states expand their SCHIP programs to include the parents and pregnant women as well.

When buying group or individual health insurance, you have the alphabet soup option of various health plans, which includes traditional, indemnity fee-for-service (FFS) plans, point-of-service (POS) plans, health maintenance organizations (HMOs), and preferred provider organizations

(PPOs). Every plan has its own significance and its own benefits. HMOs, PPOs, and POS plans are categorized as the “managed care” plans, which focus on gainful medical care.

Fee for service (FFS) coverage, also known as traditional insurance, provides the greatest convenience in exchange for higher out-of-pocket costs and greater premiums. The merits of the FFS plans include the absence of networks, you are able to select the doctors and hospitals of your choice, no permission is required for visiting any specialist, and there’s no need to initiate a visit with a primary care physician (PCP) if you want to visit a specialist of your own choice. A majority of the FFS plans have a cap, which is the maximum amount you will have to pay for medical bills in a single year. A cap is reached when all of your out-of-pocket costs/expenditures (deductibles and co-insurance) total a specific amount. The insurance company is then responsible for paying 100% of anything that is reasonable and customary. The cap amount is exclusive of your premium.

The disadvantage of the FFS system is the deductible (somewhere between $500 and $1,500). This must be met before the insurance company will pay on any claims. After that, doctors are refunded 80 percent of the bill and you are responsible for 20%. Your responsibility is termed “co-insurance.” You may even have to pre-pay for medical services and then submit bills for reimbursement. In order to obtain reimbursement, you are required to complete forms and give them to the insurer, or find a physician willing to have his office submit them on your behalf. Receipts for medications and other medical costs must also be retained. FFS plans make payments for "reasonable and customary" medical costs. If your doctor charges an extraordinarily higher fee, the difference will have to be paid from your pocket. Furthermore, your deductible doesn't include all of your health expenses; it covers only the services that fall under the policy.

HMOs are regarded as the being the least expensive health insurance plans in terms of premiums, and are also considered to have the least amount of flexibility. The sole aim of an HMO is to decrease health care costs by bringing more defensive and preventative health services into play. HMOs are intended to protect the individual's health, along with offering sufficient medical care when a disease or illness is experienced. The merits of the HMOs are that they provide comparatively less co-payments and have the least amount of paperwork. They provide coverage for several defensive-care and health-enhancement plans. Generally, there is an extensive selection of doctors and hospitals on HMO networks. Usually smaller payments (or co-payments) are made that fall somewhere between $15 and $20 per visit to a physician (under the network established by the HMO). In general, essential health services with an HMO include physician services, outpatient services, medical care, temporary mental health services and outpatient/

inpatient emergency room appointments.

The demerits of the HMO are that a primary care physician (PCP) must be selected, and you are required to visit in-network doctors; otherwise you have to pay for a greater part of the bill, or sometimes even the entire bill. The management of the health care expenses, under the doctor's guidance, is linked to the HMO and greater health care expenses detract from the physician's salary. Getting a recommendation from your PCP for visiting a specialist is necessary. In case lab testing is required and the patient uses an out-of-network lab, the reimbursement may be denied. If your regular physician abandons the HMO program, you are responsible for finding another physician in the plan.

POS plans are known for their flexibility and convenience when compared to the HMOs. However, they too want you to choose a primary care physician. A POS plan incorporates a combination of the care feature of an HMO with the preference aspect of customary medical insurance. The POS plan positions a system of health care providers who are responsible for the treatment of plan members, for a lesser fee or co-payment, however when any kind of sickness or mishap is experienced, the patient has the right to opt for a doctor outside the system. At that time, reimbursement may have to be negotiated.

The advantage of the POS plan is that you have the right to select a doctor outside the system and even obtain coverage — but the amount covered will be considerably less when compared to visiting a physician inside the plan's system. POS plans are intended to provide extra-defensive care and welfare services, including workshops on the elimination of smoking, and health club concessions. One disadvantage is the necessity to choose a PCP.

PPOs provide a financial incentive to all of its policy holders — affordable co-payments (also known as co-pays) — to be inside the group's system of practitioners.

The PPO's advantage is that, for a usual office visit, the regular co-payment is around $10 within standard timings, and no permission is required to visit any specialist of your choice, on the condition that the doctor is a member of the network. A PPO disadvantages is that when visiting an out-of-network doctor, you may be required to make payments for the whole bill from your own pocket and then submit it for repayment.

Your first step in researching health coverage is to look at coverage options and price quotes online or to contact an insurance agent of your choice. Frequently, the PPO deductible is the highest among small to mid-size employers, and this cost is rising. Check if you have to make payments for a deductible if you decide to go outside the network, or need to pay the difference between the fees of network doctors and out-of-network doctors. You may be charged greater co-payments than what is determined on the plan if the physician charges more than what is measured as "reasonable and customary."

Your personal health insurance requirements must be discussed with your agent. Analyze all the factors when thinking about the coverage you must opt for. Ask questions like: Is your doctor a part of the network? How much will a regular physical exam cost? In case of hospitalization, what costs will I incur? Is it inclusive of well-child visits? Is there a need for prescription drug coverage? Should I obtain dental coverage as well?

CHAPTER 14

Alternative Care

Alternative medicine, previously a practice championed only by chiropractors, acupuncturists, and herbalists, is now mainstream due to positive outcomes shown by dedicated research. Many physicians are seeking further training in certain aspects of alternative medicine because of the frustration and failure of traditional approaches. For many patients who suffer from syndromes, such as fibromyalgia, chronic fatigue, and some auto-immune disorders, there is no traditional pill or procedure available to help or cure them. For years, in my own practice, I have recognized pain patterns that no Western traditional medicine approach could explain. This frustrating dilemma led me to the study of acupuncture, in which I became board-certified. Eastern philosophies, such as acupuncture, which is many thousands of years old, fully explain the syndromes and "atypical pain patterns," otherwise not diagnosed or managed by our traditional medical system. By integrating Eastern and alternative approaches to the existing traditional approaches, a much broader spectrum of patients can be diagnosed and successfully treated. The purpose of this chapter is to explain some of the imbalances and issues that can play a role in chronic pain and then to discuss some of the alternative options for therapy.

During the last few years, some impressive integrative medicine representatives have managed to gain a foothold as medical experts with a variety of opinions and approaches. Mehmet C. Oz, M.D., a New York City cardiologist, focuses on keeping patients healthier by making lifestyle and dietary changes, thus weaning them from prescription drug dependence. His practice combines Western techniques such as minimally invasive surgery, with the Eastern approaches of meditation and massage.

Dr. John Sarno, professor of physical medicine and rehabilitation at New York University, has received great exposure and notoriety after writing a book entitled, The Mind/Body Prescription. He believes in the power of the mind and its ability to trigger imbalances in the body which manifest as pain. For example, though the patient's perception and symptoms of back pain are real, he believes that the mind is often more the culprit than abnormalities in low back anatomy. The mind triggers muscle tension, nerve hypersensitivity, and circulatory changes, perceived by the mind as pain. In his theory, the mind's creation of pain symptoms is meant to distract the individual from the real issues of tension, anxiety, or anger. This, of course, is an approach under much debate. He now has published many books which support the postulate that most back pain is triggered by psychological factors instead of those of physiologic origin.

Aside from lifestyle and psychological reasons for disrupting the body's fine balance and producing pain, there are many medical issues such as infectious agents, environmental toxin exposure, and certain disease states that can also be responsible for pain. It has long been known that if the body is not functioning at all levels (including energy, hormones and thoughts) it can't function optimally. The goal of integrative practitioners is to walk a patient through a very gradual, detailed assessment and treatment process. The systems that are most commonly evaluated and treated include the GI tract and hormonal assessment (including the thyroid), detoxification and nutrients. For example, if a patient does not have an "intact" gastrointestinal (GI) tract, there can be a very high incidence of headaches and joint pain due to immune reactions. Up to 75% of the immune system for the body is based in the GI tract. Additionally, half of the detoxification system for the entire body is based in the gut. With highly-sensitive testing, it has been found that most people have an overload of bacteria and yeast in the colon. Over time, the lining of the GI tract becomes inflamed and large spaces open up between the intestinal cells. These large spaces have led to the descriptive name, "leaky gut." The open spaces allow for toxins and food particles that are normally too big to enter to the bloodstream to pass through. The liver then becomes overwhelmed and the detoxification needs are heightened, thus putting a strain on nutrient stores and causing depletion. Patients become even more symptomatic as they get treated with medications for the resultant headaches, joint pain, auto-immune processes, etc., because medications require breakdown and metabolism by the liver. Often, a toxic metabolite is produced that the body can't dispose of, leading to more pain and other symptoms.

There are also multiple studies in the scientific literature on the effects of hormones for pain control as well as for numerous other symptoms. In women, symptoms of menopause can start to occur up to 15 years prior to cessation of the menstrual cycle. There are natural hormones that are biologically identical to what the body makes, and they are the only safe way to replace hormones. Different hormones will help with specific symptoms. The main hormones are estrogen, progesterone, testosterone, DHEA, and cortisol. Estrogen is responsible for greater retention of memory, helps mood, decreases blood pressure, alters skin collagen, and has many more actions. If progesterone is deficient, there is a significant increase in pain and inflammation (as well as anxiety and depression, which can increase susceptibility to chronic pain). Patients with progesterone deficiencies also have a high incidence of insomnia. Testosterone can help with sex drive, muscle mass, and motivation, among other things. DHEA replacement decreases joint pain, receptors for pain, and improves one's quality of life. Cortisol is involved in stress, sleep, the immune system, and is involved with all of the other hormones as well. These hormone levels can be measured and with salivary testing.

There are many different hormonal needs, and recommendations must be customized for each individual patient. An imbalance in thyroid hormone can affect every metabolic function in the body. It regulates energy, growth, tissue repair, heat production, and other hormones, and has many other functions as well. Furthermore, many of the standard tests used by physicians to test thyroid levels are unable to detect a large percentage of patients with under-functioning or subclinical disease. Natural hormonal therapies can be prescribed, and with the help of a compounding pharmacist, a patient can be on the path to hormonal balance. Often, once balanced, patients will have improvements in multiple symptoms that range from the expected relief of post menopausal complaints to weight loss and the resolution of chronic pain.

Detoxification is also helpful with multiple symptoms such as fatigue, headaches, joint pain, and muscle weakness. Many environmental toxins, such as heavy metals, plasticides, pesticides, etc., can cause disease. Unfortunately, these chemicals have become ubiquitous in our air, water, and food supply. In fact, a surprising and frightening study showed that even Inuit Indian mothers living in the Arctic have a multitude of modern chemicals in their breast milk. These toxins can be handled by the body for a period of time, but they can eventually overwhelm the system and cause disease. Free radical exposure from the environment causes oxidation which leads to various diseases and requires very high doses of antioxidants to neutralize them. Treatment remedies such as oral detoxification protocols, colonics, and infrared saunas can help to decrease the toxic load, optimize health, and decrease a multitude of symptomatology.

Proper nutrition is imperative for the treatment and prevention of disease. Various committees have come up with guidelines that typically are not stringent enough to insure optimal health. Additionally each person has individual needs for vitamins and minerals. Medications, stress, soil depletion, toxins, age, and genetics may influence a particular person's needs. We also know that people with better nutritional, dietary, and exercise habits, live longer and healthier lives. In Dr. Pamela Smith's book, What You Must Know About Vitamins, Minerals, Herbs, and More, she reviews each nutrient, the recommended doses for optimal health, causes of deficiency, symptoms of both deficiency and excess, and how to get the right dose through both food and nutritional supplementation. There are also tests that can tell which specific nutrients a patient is deficient in and allow his physician to come up with a plan individualized for his needs. This can help even patients with genetic predispositions for certain diseases. For example, it is now known that even if you have a particular gene for Alzheimers disease, it depends on the environment (i.e. stress, toxins and nutrients) that the gene is subject to whether or not the actual disease develops.

Therefore, eating a good and balanced diet is important to maximize your nutritional benefit. Diets high in calories and fats, along with excessive body weight are linked to heart disease, diabetes, cancer, and joint degeneration. Adjusting your diet to include more fruits and vegetables will help minimize this risk. We are inundated with dietary supplements at health food stores; some of the more common agents possibly helpful to reduce pain and inflammation include the following: coenzyme Q10, which helps your body produce energy (ATP) and also functions as an antioxidant; echinacea, which boosts the immune system; flax seed oil, which decreases inflammation and may reduce the risk of heart attacks and stroke; garlic, which may reduce cholesterol and the risk of heart attack and stroke; glucosamine, which may decrease osteoarthritis; lycopenes (found in vegetables), that are antioxidants and may reduce risk of cancers and heart disease; melatonin, which may aid in sleep; and St. John's wort, which may improve depression and aid in wound healing.

"Chiropractic" is a word derived from the Greek words Cheiros and Praktikos meaning "Hand Practice." It is a healing practice that has been used for nearly 5000 years. Hippocrates (60-375 BC), one of the fathers of medicine said, "In disease, always look to the spine first." The chiropractic approach is largely based upon the assumption that a misaligned bone, referred to as a "subluxation," causes a distortion in nerves located in close proximity to the bone, leading to pain and disease. Chiropractors treat these subluxations through manipulation, and thereby attempt to restore proper alignment. If subluxations persist, they can eventually result in pain by affecting the bones, ligaments, discs, muscles, and nerves. Often, multiple adjustments are needed since the locked joints, with altered tendon and ligament lengths, tend to want to return to their malaligned state before adjusting to their more properly aligned anatomy.

Massage therapy is another manual therapy, but focuses on decreasing overall muscle tension, not on addressing bone subluxations. This is accomplished through soothing manipulation of the muscles and overlying skin, thereby aiding in increasing the parasympathetic nervous system tone (rest and digest) and decreasing the sympathetic nervous system tone (fight or flight). Sympathetic nervous system activation increases muscle tension, while massage therapy decreases it. By minimizing sympathetic tone which entails the emotion of stress, pain is relieved and one's sense of self-esteem and well-being is markedly improved.

Acupuncture is an ancient Oriental treatment for disease states and pain and is accomplished by the insertion of hair-thin needles into certain meridians or energy pathways located throughout the body. As compared to the relative infancy of Western medicine, this technique has been in existence for over two thousand years. The concept behind acupuncture lies in the restoration in balance of yin and yang within the body, thereby allowing "Chi," or energy, to flow freely and harmoniously. When chi flows freely, the person is healthy. When a person is sick or injured, then there is an obstruction to the flow of chi, and stagnation occurs. Sometimes this is referred to as "phlegm", which can accumulate along certain meridian or energy points. Examination often reveals these areas to be tender or swollen. When needles are inserted into these stagnation points, energy is introduced into the meridian pathway system by gently twisting the needle, by adding electrical current, or the application of heat. A dozen or more needles are usually needed to alter the flow of chi; this can be conceptualized as rewiring or bypassing a faulty electrical circuit. When needles are in the correct location, the patient often describes sensations of pleasant warmth, heaviness, or tingling spreading throughout the area as the chi begins to flow again. Many of these needle insertion sites are identical to Western medicines' trigger point, and ligament and tendon attachment locations.

From a Western viewpoint, there may be one of many possible mechanisms to explain the acupuncture benefit. Acupuncture may cause the central nervous system to release pain–suppressing neurotransmitters; it may also cause the release of our own endorphins, or naturally-occurring morphine, known to be associated with the "runners high." Acupuncture may also influence the body's ability to regulate blood flow and temperature, probably through changes in the autonomic or sympathetic nervous system.

Nambudripad's Allergy Elimination Techniques (NAET) is a non-invasive, drug-free method that helps balance energy in the body. It operates on a principle similar to acupuncture, viewing energy imbalances as causative of health issues, including pain. NAET views allergies – including environmental and food allergies, as the mechanism causing this imbalance. Once the allergy is removed via a series of non-invasive, desensitization procedures, then balance and wellness are restored.

Cognitive Behavioral Therapy (CBT) is a form of psychosocial therapy used in the treatment of many different disease states including pain. The theory of CBT is that maladaptive thought processes trigger negative behaviors and emotions which, in turn, have been associated with increased pain scores. By increasing awareness of these negative behaviors and emotions, you can more readily change them into positive healthy ones. This will increase your contentment with life and result in decreased pain.

Common tools used in CBT include keeping a written journal of the daily events and their associated emotions, actions, and pain scores. Cognitive reversal is another tool. The patient relates a stressful situation to the therapist, who then helps to reinterpret the events from a healthier and more productive viewpoint. Systemic sensitization is a tool whereby the patient imagines an uncomfortable and stressful situation. The therapist assists the patient in relaxing, thereby desensitizing the patient after many repetitive exposures. With all the CBT techniques altering the associated anxiety and depression seen with chronic pain, many patients will have improved quality of life, greater function, and reduced pain scores.

Biofeedback is yet another tool to decrease the body's response to stress and associated pain. This is accomplished by using your mind to control your body's physiological responses, resulting in improved self-esteem and a feeling of well-being. Pain associated stressful disorders often responds to this modality including anxiety, migraines, teeth grinding (TMJ), and fibromyalgia. This technique is accomplished through the application of several body sensors, thus increasing your physiologic awareness. These sensors may include brain electroencephalograms (EEG), blood pressure, heart rate, electromyography (EMG) for muscle tension, skin temperature, and sweat production. By visualizing these changes, you become more adept at recognizing the role of stress and pain on the body. The next step is altering the pathological responses on the monitor, assisted via auditory or visual monitor cues, which give feedback and a sense of positive reinforcement. This approach has improved self-control, self-confidence, and has reduced stress with its associated pain. This form of mind-body medicine complements many other similar techniques to control pain.

Weight loss is another key factor in addressing pain. Obesity is a known epidemic in the United States with 45% of adults over the age of 60 being obese. Associated with the obesity is a decrease in physical activity, resulting in a lack of muscle tone needed for skeletal support. Obesity puts excessive wear and tear not only on the spine, but also on the muscles and joints, causing a diffuse pain syndrome which surgery, injections, physical therapy, and medications fail to resolve. The body is not designed to successfully carry around that excessive weight and breakdown quickly occurs, especially after the age of 50. I have many patients whose pain is so tightly related to their weight that a gain of just 3 pounds causes knee or back pain; a 3 pound weight loss will quickly resolve their discomfort. Besides pain, other medical illnesses are drastically increased in incidence by being even 10% overweight. These include hypertension, diabetes, heart disease, and strokes, to name a few. When treating obesity and chronic pain, dietary consultation and counseling with strict guidelines is essential; weight loss attempt without this professional support is often futile. I have patients keep a daily log of intake, and they quickly become amazed to learn how poorly they control their diet.

We are all guilty of this, some of us worse than others; you know who you are. After viewing the dietary log, patients quickly reduce non-essential eating and progress positively to gradual and satisfactory weight loss with subsequent reduction of pain.

Depression is a mental illness that is commonly seen in the chronic pain population, each illness exacerbating the other. Depression and pain also share some of the same neurotransmitters, namely serotonin. Decreased serotonin levels, therefore, are seen in depression; it is an imbalance targeted by many therapies. Vitamin B6 is made into serotonin and extra doses may increase serotonin levels. Foods containing elevated vitamin B6 levels include nuts, fish, liver, and turkey. Vitamin B6 is broken down into the chemical tryptophan; hence it is another agent which can be augmented by consuming foods high in its content. Milk, meat, and cheese contain high levels of tryptophan. Nutritional counseling can therefore play a critical role with chronic pain patients, especially when chronic pain is associated with depression and obesity.

This book should remain in a convenient location after reading as a reference. I hope it answers many of your common and daily pain concerns, allowing you maximum enjoyment and comfort in your life in the absence of pain. If I have shared some knowledge to improve your life and understanding of this "dis-ease" known as pain, then I am most grateful.

About the book cover and artist:

Stephen M. Saff is an architect, furniture designer, and artist who lives and works in the Washington DC area. He comes from an art background; his father Donald Saff spent most of his professional life collaborating with world-class artists to produce limited editions and cutting-edge works of art. Growing up in this environment had a profound effect on Stephen's early teen years and led him to eventually pursue a professional career as an architect. Architecture for him was, at first, a great profession for expressing his artistic passion, but in the last ten years he started exploring making art as a new, creative venue. This particular artistic venue gave him greater license to pursue his ideas, unencumbered by clients and functional constraints. His biggest artistic influence came from the artist Robert Rauschenberg, one of numerous artists that had collaborated with his father over the course of some thirty-plus years. Rauschenberg explored the world of photographic images, the play of images when combined with a multitude of techniques, layering, and processes, and created an amazing dialectic of new meanings and visual associations. It is this type of layering of images and interplay of these images that became the backbone of a process and visual language that Stephen is exploring in his own work.

The book cover is an assemblage of images that relate to the body, mind, and senses, the physical display of pleasure and pain, and the mechanics and mechanism of all the body systems that carry and produce the physical and mental state of man. The image of the poppy flower is an obvious connection to the use of nature's opiate, used historically in medicine to treat pain. The two main images of the man and woman are a play on the dichotomy of pain and joy, or lack of pain. The man is in physical and mental pain; this image bleeds into the CT scan-like image of the human head with the brain shown as green and sickly while the rest of the body is shown as more red and yellowish. The woman is free from pain and is in a state of bliss and elation; she appears to be in an almost euphoric state. Since colors are often used to describe or evoke an emotional and physical state, the colors were manipulated accordingly to produce different emotions relative to different forms of physical and emotional body and mind states. On the back of the cover, again the same image of the man is used, but the color is changed to demonstrate a change in the level of pain. Faded behind this image is a diagram of the human body, with the attached graphic lines indicating different body anatomic and neurologic locations. One would see this type of graphic image in a doctor's office or at an acupuncture treatment center.

All these representational images are entwined and interconnected just like all the parts of the human body, whether physical or mental. The images are interconnected and interlaced into a collage to reflect this theme of different physical and mental states of being.

INDEX[1*]

A

B

D

E

F

G

H

I

M

N

O

P

Q

R

S

T

U

V

W

X

Y